Environmental Disasters and Individuals' Emergency Preparedness: In the Perspective of Psychology and Behavior

Environmental Disasters and Individuals' Emergency Preparedness: In the Perspective of Psychology and Behavior

Editors

Yuxiang Hong
Ziqiang Han
Jong-Suk Kim
Joo-Heon Lee

MDPI • Basel • Beijing • Wuhan • Barcelona • Belgrade • Manchester • Tokyo • Cluj • Tianjin

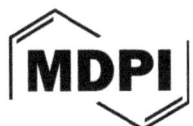

Editors

Yuxiang Hong
School of Management
Hangzhou Dianzi University
Hangzhou
China

Ziqiang Han
School of Political Science and
Public Administration
Shandong University
Qingdao
China

Jong-Suk Kim
Department of Hydrology and
Water Resources
Wuhan University
Wuhan
China

Joo-Heon Lee
Civil Engineering Department
Joongbu University
Gyeonggi-DO
Korea, South

Editorial Office
MDPI
St. Alban-Anlage 66
4052 Basel, Switzerland

This is a reprint of articles from the Special Issue published online in the open access journal *International Journal of Environmental Research and Public Health* (ISSN 1660-4601) (available at: www. mdpi.com/journal/ijerph/special_issues/environmental_disasters).

For citation purposes, cite each article independently as indicated on the article page online and as indicated below:

LastName, A.A.; LastName, B.B.; LastName, C.C. Article Title. *Journal Name* **Year**, *Volume Number*, Page Range.

ISBN 978-3-0365-3235-6 (Hbk)
ISBN 978-3-0365-3234-9 (PDF)

© 2022 by the authors. Articles in this book are Open Access and distributed under the Creative Commons Attribution (CC BY) license, which allows users to download, copy and build upon published articles, as long as the author and publisher are properly credited, which ensures maximum dissemination and a wider impact of our publications.

The book as a whole is distributed by MDPI under the terms and conditions of the Creative Commons license CC BY-NC-ND.

Contents

About the Editors vii

Preface to "Environmental Disasters and Individuals' Emergency Preparedness: In the Perspective of Psychology and Behavior" ix

Kaijing Xue, Shili Guo, Yi Liu, Shaoquan Liu and Dingde Xu
Social Networks, Trust, and Disaster-Risk Perceptions of Rural Residents in a Multi-Disaster Environment: Evidence from Sichuan, China
Reprinted from: *Int. J. Environ. Res. Public Health* **2021**, *18*, 2106, doi:10.3390/ijerph18042106 . . . 1

Hainan Huang, Weifan Chen, Tian Xie, Yaoyao Wei, Ziqing Feng and Weijiong Wu
The Impact of Individual Behaviors and Governmental Guidance Measures on Pandemic-Triggered Public Sentiment Based on System Dynamics and Cross-Validation
Reprinted from: *Int. J. Environ. Res. Public Health* **2021**, *18*, 4245, doi:10.3390/ijerph18084245 . . . 27

Ziyi Wang, Ziqiang Han, Lin Liu and Shaobin Yu
Place Attachment and Household Disaster Preparedness: Examining the Mediation Role of Self-Efficacy
Reprinted from: *Int. J. Environ. Res. Public Health* **2021**, *18*, 5565, doi:10.3390/ijerph18115565 . . . 53

Teng Zhao, Yuchen Zhang, Chao Wu and Qiang Su
Will Anti-Epidemic Campus Signals Affect College Students' Preparedness in the Post-COVID-19 Era?
Reprinted from: *Int. J. Environ. Res. Public Health* **2021**, *18*, 9276, doi:10.3390/ijerph18179276 . . . 67

Ning Zhang, Zichen Wang, Lan Zhang and Xiao Yang
Assessment of Water Resources Carrying Risk and the Coping Behaviors of the Government and the Public
Reprinted from: *Int. J. Environ. Res. Public Health* **2021**, *18*, 7693, doi:10.3390/ijerph18147693 . . . 81

Yingnan Ma, Wei Zhu, Huan Zhang, Pengxia Zhao, Yafei Wang and Qiujie Zhang
The Factors Affecting Volunteers' Willingness to Participate in Disaster Preparedness
Reprinted from: *Int. J. Environ. Res. Public Health* **2021**, *18*, 4141, doi:10.3390/ijerph18084141 . . . 101

Huihui Wang, Jiaqing Zhao, Ying Wang and Yuxiang Hong
Study on the Formation Mechanism of Medical and Health Organization Staff's Emergency Preparedness Behavioral Intention: From the Perspective of Psychological Capital
Reprinted from: *Int. J. Environ. Res. Public Health* **2021**, *18*, 8246, doi:10.3390/ijerph18168246 . . . 111

About the Editors

Yuxiang Hong

Dr. Yuxiang Hong is an associate professor at School of Management, Hangzhou Dianzi University, China. His previous experience includes working as a visiting scholar at Utrecht University (2012-2013) and University of Plymouth (2018-2019). His research focuses on the interdisciplinary studies combining environment, human capital, technology, and risk. Research areas include: human aspect of security, emergency preparedness, risk communication, environmental psychology.

Ziqiang Han

Ziqiang Han is a full professor and the executive director of the Center for Risk Governance and Emergency Management at the School of Political Science and Public Administration, Shandong University. Dr. Han obtains his Ph.D. degree from the Disaster Science and Management program at the Disaster Research Center, University of Delaware, and his current research focuses on disaster preparedness, comprehensive school safety, and urban resilience.

Jong-Suk Kim

Prof. Jong-Suk Kim works at the Department of Hydrology and Water Resources, Wuhan University, China. His research work focuses on diagnostic analysis and assessment methodologies to understand hydroclimatic change, nonstationarity in hydroclimatic extremes, emergency preparedness behavior for natural disasters, and an integrated view of climate and hydrologic variability and changes.

Joo-Heon Lee

Joo-Heon Lee obtained his Ph.D. from Kyung Hee University, Korea. Now Dr. Lee is a professor of the Civil Engineering Department at Joongbu University and the vice-Chair of UNESCO IHP Korea National Committee. His research area primarily focuses on drought (monitoring and forecasting), climate change (vulnerability and adaptation), hydrometeorology, ecohydrology, hydrologic extremes (flood and drought), and remote sensing.

Preface to "Environmental Disasters and Individuals' Emergency Preparedness: In the Perspective of Psychology and Behavior"

Environmental disasters are becoming more frequent. These disasters not only include the most common natural disasters, but also include man-made disasters, such as public health, accident disasters, etc., which have caused greater damage to human society and cities. Because of the limitations of a single government-led model in emergency response, the emergency preparedness of communities, families and individuals are more important. In particular, the emergency preparedness psychology and behavior of individuals directly determine whether or not they can effectively protect themselves and their families in the first time of disaster. This Special Issue focuses on environmental disasters and individuals' emergency preparedness in the perspective of psychology and behavior.

Yuxiang Hong, Ziqiang Han, Jong-Suk Kim, Joo-Heon Lee
Editors

Social Networks, Trust, and Disaster-Risk Perceptions of Rural Residents in a Multi-Disaster Environment: Evidence from Sichuan, China

Kaijing Xue [1,2], Shili Guo [3], Yi Liu [4], Shaoquan Liu [1,*] and Dingde Xu [5,*]

1. Institute of Mountain Hazards and Environment, Chinese Academy of Sciences, #9, Block 4, Renminnan Road, Chengdu 610041, China; kaijingxue@imde.ac.cn
2. Institute of Mountain Hazards and Environment, University of Chinese Academy of Sciences, No. 19A Yuquan Road, Beijing 100049, China
3. China Western Economic Research Center, Southwestern University of Finance and Economics, Chengdu 610074, China; guoshili@swufe.edu.cn
4. College of Management of Sichuan Agricultural University, Chengdu 611130, China; lyx1@stu.sicau.edu.cn
5. Sichuan Center for Rural Development Research, College of Management, Sichuan Agricultural University, 211 Huimin Road, Wenjiang District, Chengdu 611130, China
* Correspondence: liushq@imde.ac.cn (S.L.); dingdexu@sicau.edu.cn (D.X.)

Abstract: Individual perception of disaster risk is not only the product of individual factors, but also the product of social interactions. However, few studies have empirically explored the correlations between rural residents' flat social networks, trust in pyramidal channels, and disaster-risk perceptions. Taking Sichuan Province—a typical disaster-prone province in China—as an example and using data from 327 rural households in mountainous areas threatened by multiple disasters, this paper measured the level of participants' disaster-risk perception in the four dimensions of possibility, threat, self-efficacy, and response efficacy. Then, the ordinary least squares method was applied to probe the correlations between social networks, trust, and residents' disaster-risk perception. The results revealed four main findings. (1) Compared with scores relating to comprehensive disaster-risk perception, participants had lower perception scores relating to possibility and threat, and higher perception scores relating to self-efficacy and response efficacy. (2) The carrier characteristics of their social networks significantly affected rural residents' perceived levels of disaster risk, while the background characteristics did not. (3) Different dimensions of trust had distinct effects on rural residents' disaster-risk perceptions. (4) Compared with social network variables, trust was more closely related to the perceived level of disaster risks, which was especially reflected in the impact on self-efficacy, response efficacy, and comprehensive perception. The findings of this study deepen understanding of the relationship between social networks, trust, and disaster-risk perceptions of rural residents in mountainous areas threatened by multiple disasters, providing enlightenment for building resilient disaster-prevention systems in the community.

Keywords: social networks; trust; risk perception; multiple disasters; China

1. Introduction

Natural disasters are events in which natural changes exceed what can be borne by humans, thereby causing harm to human society and the economy [1]. Natural disasters mainly include geophysical disasters—such as earthquakes and volcanoes—and disasters caused by weather or climate—such as floods, storms, and landslides. In recent years, with changes in global climate and increases in the scope and intensity of human activities, the frequency and degree of harm of various natural disasters have risen significantly, which has had far-reaching impacts on global economic and social development. In 2019, nearly 1900 natural disasters displaced 24.9 million people in 140 countries and regions, causing an estimated 137 billion dollars in economic losses according to the Internal Displacement

Monitoring Centre and the Swiss Re Institute [2,3]. It is worth noting that Asia was among the most affected regions, both in terms of the number of people affected and the economic losses caused.

Mountainous areas, in addition to being regions with frequent natural disasters, are also characterized by chain reactions and mass occurrence of disasters. Residents in mountainous areas, especially rural residents, live in scattered communities with weak economic foundations and insufficient awareness of disaster prevention, all of which lead to more severe disaster threats [4,5]. China is a mountainous country: mountains account for 69% of the total land area and 45% of the population live in mountainous areas [6–8]. China is also a disaster-prone country [9]. From 2010 to 2018, about 244 million people were affected by natural disasters in China, resulting in direct economic losses of about 3520.4 billion yuan [10]. These disasters included 129 earthquakes with a magnitude of five or above and 117,299 geological disasters such as landslides and debris flows.

In regions where multiple disaster risks coexist and there is a risk of serious harm, effective risk management has become a challenge for governments and academia. However, previous studies on disaster-risk management have primarily focused on single types of disasters such as earthquakes, floods, or landslides [11–13]; there has been little attention paid to situations where the risk of multiple disasters coexists. Furthermore, the research areas were mainly in developed countries such as the USA and in Europe [14–16], with relatively few in developing countries or in Asia.

Many empirical studies have shown that residents' risk perceptions will prompt them to take active risk mitigation actions [17,18]. For example, Miceli et al. [19] investigated the relationship between flood risk perceptions and prevention preparedness of residents in the northern Italian mountains, and found that residents' anxiety and perceptions of flood-risk possibility were positively correlated with prevention preparedness. Xu et al. [20] explored the correlation between landslide risk perception and prevention behavior and found that residents' perceived levels of the possibility and threat had significant and positive effects on active disaster preparedness. As disaster-risk perception plays an important role in the construction of disaster prevention and reduction systems at the family level, theories relating to disaster-risk perception are attracting increasing attention from scholars and managers. Disaster-risk perception evaluates the levels of an individual's impression and awareness of disaster risks. Based on different goals, scholars have measured disaster-risk perceptions from different dimensions, including the possibility, impact, severity, controllability, and fear of disaster risks [19,21–23]. However, as the final point of disaster-risk management is the level of disaster prevention and mitigation activity, considering only how people feel about the disaster event itself fails to closely combine residents' risk perceptions with corresponding adaptive behaviors.

On the basis of previous disaster-risk perception studies, some scholars have undertaken additional exploration of the relationships among residents' self-efficacy, response efficacy, risk perceptions, and individual adaptive actions [17,24–26]. In essence, the intrinsic meaning of residents' self-efficacy and response efficacy for disaster risks is the perception evaluation that they use to solve and deal with the disaster threats, respectively [27,28]. Therefore, in a broad sense, residents' self-efficacy and response efficacy for disaster risks also belong to residents' perceptions of disaster risks. Theoretically, it is feasible to integrate these two dimensions and disaster-risk perceptions into generalized disaster-risk perceptions. This study considered that generalized disaster-risk perception should include the perception evaluation of the disaster risk event itself as well as the degree of mitigation that can be achieved. However, few scholars have explored the integration of these two aspects; therefore, there is still a need to measure residents' levels of generalized disaster-risk perception so that these can be more closely connected to residents' adaptive actions.

In terms of the factors that influence residents' disaster-risk perceptions, many studies have focused on the impact of socio-economic factors of individuals and families—such as gender, age, education, duration of residence, family population, etc.; disaster experience—

including whether they had experienced a disaster, the number of times of disaster experience, etc.; and response preparation—such as building reinforcement, disaster insurance, etc. [20,29–33]. Social networks are a form of social resource that can provide people with social support [34]. Especially in mountainous rural areas with relatively isolated information, social networks can become the carrier of disaster-risk information, affecting individuals' thinking and judgment regarding disaster risks, and thus continuously adjusting residents' perceptions of disaster risks [35–38]. Therefore, residents' perceptions of disaster risks are not only the product of personal factors, but also the product of interpersonal and social interaction processes. However, previous academic research has mostly analyzed social networks as a part of social capital and social support, and there has been little empirical research on the correlation between social networks and disaster-risk perceptions [39,40]; that is, previous research approaches have failed to characterize social networks as carriers. Therefore, the challenge of measuring social networks reasonably, according to their characteristics, and then determining relationships between social networks and disaster-risk perceptions is worth exploring. In addition, inside the community, residents get some services from the community management organization and are also bound by it to a certain extent. Previous studies have shown that residents' trust in community management organizations is a key factor affecting their perceptions of disaster risks [32,40,41]. In fact, the information and safeguard measures confirmed and released by management organizations generally come from higher-level formal organizations with high authority and credibility, indicating that residents' trust in community management organizations is trust in formal pyramidal channels [42]. However, the information and the support contained in social networks are more accessible but less exact, which shows the informal flat characteristics of social networks [43]. Accordingly, the effects of these two different types of channels on residents' perceptions of disaster risks are another question worth exploring.

In this context, taking Sichuan Province—a typical disaster-prone province in China—as an example, and selecting residents in mountainous areas threatened by earthquakes, landslides, mountain torrents, and other disasters as the research object, this study measured the level of the interviewees' disaster-risk perception in terms of the four dimensions of possibility, threat, self-efficacy, and response efficacy. Furthermore, the ordinary least squares method was used to probe the correlations and differences between social networks, trust in community management organizations, and residents' disaster-risk perceptions to enrich the relevant research and provide reference for the government to formulate disaster prevention and mitigation measures.

2. Material and Methods

2.1. Research Area

Located in southwest China, Sichuan Province is dominated by hills and mountains which account for about 90% of the total area [44–46]. Sichuan is a typical disaster-prone province in China. Apart from earthquakes, there are also geological disasters such as landslides and mud-rock flows. From 2008 to 2018, 19 earthquakes of magnitude five or above occurred in Sichuan province, causing a total of 460,000 casualties and 856.8 billion yuan of direct economic losses, accounting for 12.34% of the total number of earthquake disasters of magnitude five and above nationwide, 95.04% of the total number of disaster casualties nationwide, and 83.13% of direct economic losses nationwide caused by disasters. Additionally, a total of 18,518 geological disasters such as landslides and mud-rock flows have occurred in Sichuan Province, causing 1390 casualties and eight billion yuan of direct economic losses; these accounted for 11.99% of all geological disasters, 16.45% of all casualties, and 13.60% of direct economic losses nationwide [10]. Of these disasters, the Wenchuan earthquake on 12 May 2008 (8 on the Richter scale) and the Lushan earthquake on 20 April 2013 (7 on the Richter scale) caused huge casualties and economic losses to local residents [23,47]. Considering the non-negligible impact of earthquake disasters on residents in multi-disaster environments, this study selected the mountainous areas hit by the Wenchuan and Lushan earthquakes as the representative research areas within Sichuan Province.

2.2. Data Sources

The data applied in this paper are primarily from a questionnaire survey conducted in July 2019 by the research group in the mountainous areas affected by the Wenchuan and Lushan earthquakes. This survey mainly investigated rural residents' sustainable livelihoods, disaster-risk perceptions, disaster-avoidance behaviors, and the construction of resilient disaster-prevention systems in the community. The survey method was a face-to-face interview of residents for about 90 min. To ensure the representativeness of the selected samples, stratified sampling and then equal probability random sampling were used to determine the research samples [48]. First, considering that the sampled counties should come from areas affected by Wenchuan and Lushan earthquakes and that at least two counties with significant differences in economic development should be selected from the same disaster area, Beichuan County and Pengzhou City (Pengzhou City is a county-level city) were selected as sample counties from 10 counties stricken by the Wenchuan Earthquake, and Baoxing County and Lushan County were selected as sample counties from six counties hit by the Lushan Earthquake. Second, according to differences in the level of economic status within a county, the distance from the center of the county and the severity of the disaster, two sample townships were chosen from each sample county. In this way, a total of eight sample towns were obtained. Third, the villages in each sample town were divided into two groups according to the number of threatened people, the difference in economic development level, and the distance from the center of the town, and one village was randomly chosen from each group. By these means, 16 sample villages were obtained in all. Finally, in each sample village, 20–23 rural households were randomly chosen with reference to a roster and random number chart [33,34,49]. According to the survey, there are a total of 1145 disaster-threatened households in 16 selected villages. Further, based on the above process, a total of 327 valid questionnaires were gained from 16 villages in 8 townships in 4 counties. The spatial locations of the sample counties and townships are shown in Figure 1.

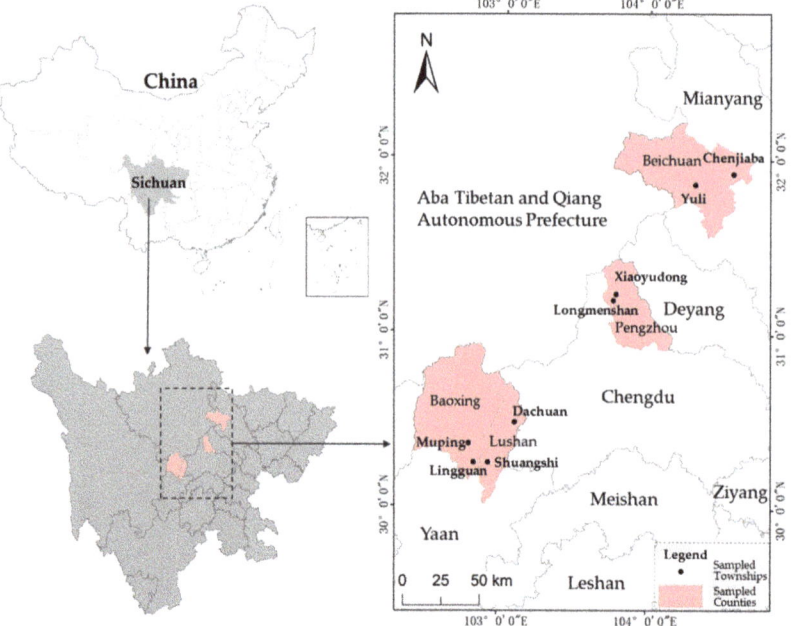

Figure 1. Distribution of sample counties and townships.

2.3. Variables and Methods

2.3.1. Selection and Definition of Model Variables

(1) Dependent variables

The dependent variables in this paper were rural residents' levels of disaster-risk perception. As mentioned above, the disaster-risk perception explored in this study was generalized, including the perception evaluation of the disaster-risk event itself and the degree of mitigation that could be achieved. Referring to the measurement methods of disaster-risk perceptions in existing literature [15,17,19,21,22,50], and combining with the data characteristics of acquired questionnaires, this paper mainly categorized entries in terms of four dimensions of disaster-risk perception—possibility, threat, self-efficacy, and response efficacy—to measure the generalized disaster-risk perception. The specific entries can be seen in Table 1. It is worth noting that, according to the survey, the types of disasters threatening residents in the study area mainly included earthquakes, landslides, debris flows, and mountain torrents. Therefore, this study relates particularly to these four types of disaster, generically. In addition, since many studies have shown that the response measures for different types of disasters are distinct, and residents' perceptions of the effectiveness of different response measures are also distinct [51–53], disaster mitigation behaviors should be suitable for the four types of disasters and choose a clear response behavior, as far as possible, to measure response efficacy. Several studies have shown that evacuation—a common behavior to avoid disasters—can effectively reduce the adverse impact of disasters on residents [33,54–56] and can be well adapted to a variety of disaster types. Therefore, the response efficacy in this study specifically refers to the degree of disaster-threat mitigation by evacuation.

Table 1. Measurement of disaster-risk perception.

Entry Code	Dimension	Item [a]	Mean	SD [b]
P1	Probability	In the next 10 years, there may be disasters near my home.	2.83	1.12
P2		I always feel that disasters will come one day.	3.08	1.32
P3		In recent years, the signs of disasters occurrence have become more and more obvious.	3.17	1.35
T1	Threat	In the next 10 years, if a disaster occurs, your house and land will be damaged.	3.84	1.14
T2		In the next 10 years, if a disaster occurs, your and your family's lives will be affected.	3.35	1.31
T3		If a disaster occurs, supplies will be cut off.	3.24	1.42
SE1	Self-efficacy	When a disaster occurs, you know the evacuation route.	4.17	1.16
SE2		You know the location of the emergency shelter in the village.	4.00	1.23
SE3		You know the disaster prevention and mitigation measures in the village.	3.28	1.30
RE1	Response efficacy	Evacuation can effectively prevent injury/death.	4.37	0.88
RE2		If I evacuate, I will effectively avoid injury/death.	4.28	0.91
RE3		Evacuation can effectively reduce the emotional and physical pain.	4.33	0.90

Note: [a] The Likert scale was used for all entries, with 1 representing complete disagreement and 5 representing complete agreement; [b] SD = standard deviation.

The specific measurement process was as follows. An internal consistency test was carried out on the entries characterizing residents' perceptions of disaster risks, with results showing that Cronbach α values corresponding to the possibility, threat, self-efficacy, response efficacy, and comprehensive perception of disaster risks were all greater than 0.60 (0.69, 0.63, 0.66, 0.81, and 0.65, respectively). This indicated that the entries were internally consistent. Then, factor analysis was used to reduce dimensionality of the disaster-risk perception entries, and four dimensions of probability, threat, self-efficacy, and response efficacy were obtained. Among these, the Kaiser–Meyer–Olkin value corresponding to factor analysis was 0.72, the P value of the Bartlett test for sphericity was 0.000 (less than 0.001), and the cumulative variance contribution rate of the four dimensions was 64.62%; all of these results indicated that the results of the factor analysis were reasonable (see Table 2 for details). Then, the min-max standardization method was adopted to convert the four-dimensional scores obtained through factor analysis into a centesimal system, according to Equation (1). Finally, the ratio of the contribution rate of single dimensional variance to the contribution rate of cumulative variance was used as the weighting to calculate residents' comprehensive perception of disaster risks according to Equation (2).

$$X_{ij}^s = \frac{x_{ij} - min(x_{ij})}{max(x_{ij}) - min(x_{ij})} \times 100 \qquad (1)$$

$$X_i^c = \sum_{j=1}^{4} (X_{ij}^s \times w_j) \qquad (2)$$

Table 2. The component matrixes of each risk perception component after rotation.

Items	Component			
	Probability	Threat	Self-Efficacy	Response Efficacy
P1	0.65	0.38	−0.09	0.09
P2	0.82	0.13	−0.22	0.05
P3	0.75	0.09	0.03	−0.11
T1	0.40	0.61	0.08	0.10
T2	0.35	0.72	0.07	0.11
T3	0.01	0.77	−0.09	−0.07
SE1	−0.13	0.19	0.70	0.17
SE2	−0.10	−0.03	0.79	0.07
SE3	0.02	−0.13	0.78	0.09
RE1	0.06	−0.03	0.09	0.86
RE2	0.02	−0.05	0.19	0.86
RE3	−0.07	0.17	0.06	0.81
Eigenvalue	1.96	1.74	1.84	2.21
Explained variance	16.37%	14.48%	15.34%	18.43%
Cumulative variance	16.37%	30.85%	46.19%	64.62%
Cronbach α	0.69	0.63	0.66	0.81

In Equations (1) and (2), X_{ij}^s is the score of the centesimal system in the j dimension of disaster-risk perception of resident i, where i (i = 1, 2, ..., 327) represents the individual residents in the sample, j (j = 1, 2, 3, 4) represents the four dimensions for measuring the disaster-risk perception of rural residents; X_i^c is the calculated score of the comprehensive perception of disaster risks of resident i; x_{ij} represents the factor comprehensive score in the j dimension of the disaster-risk perception of resident i; $min(x_{ij})$ represents the minimum value of the factor comprehensive score in the j dimension of disaster-risk perceptions of rural residents; $max(x_{ij})$ represents the maximum value of the factor comprehensive score in the j dimension of disaster-risk perception of rural residents and w_j refers to the ratio of the contribution rate of single dimensional variance to the contribution rate of cumulative variance.

(2) Focal variables

The social networks of rural residents were a core independent variable in this study. In the field of sociology research, there are usually two perspectives to discuss social networks. First, the social network is regarded as an analytical tool, with which the relationship between actors and the environment can be clarified [57]. The second is to view the social network as a social structure made up of relationships between actors, and the relationships contained in social networks become the research object [58]. Specifically, in this study, the social network was defined as the collection of nodes (typically referred to as social actors) together with a set of ties (typically known as social relations) that connect pairs of nodes [59], which can provide social support and share risk for people [60]. At present, there is not a recognized research paradigm for the study of social network, and scholars have distinguishing emphases on the study of social network. At the micro level, some scholars explored the structural characteristics of the internal nodes of social networks; some focused on the roles of strong and weak ties [61,62]; and some were concerned about the differences in social relations between different identities (such as kinship, friendship, acquaintanceship, etc.) [63]. Different from the above studies, since the data at each node were limited, the scale of this study was slightly expanded, that is, it considered individuals' social networks as a whole. In light of the measurement of social capital at the individual level [39,64,65], indicators representing the overall background characteristics of the social network can be selected as the scale, density, heterogeneity, centrality, and quality of the social network. In addition, social capital represents potential resources, which are in the network of personal relationships. In comparison to social capital, the advantage of the social network is that it can express the actual carrier function of social relations. In addition, Borgatti and Li [66] have shown that both "hard" types of ties (e.g., materials and money flows) and "soft" types of ties (e.g., friendships and sharing-of-information) are crucial (and mutually embedded) in the supply chain context. To sum up, taking into account the background characteristics of social networks as well as their characteristics as carriers, and referring to research on the measurement of social networks by Scherer and Cho [67], Heaney and Israel [60], Reininger, Rahbar, Lee, Chen, Alam, Pope, and Adams [39], and Jones, Faas, Murphy, Tobin, and Mccarty [37], this study categorized residents' social network variables in terms of background characteristics and carrier characteristics. Further, consider the characteristics of the data obtained, background features are characterized by the scale and heterogeneity of the network, and carrier features are measured by their substance and information transfer functions.

Specifically, Chinese New Year is the most important festival every year for all Chinese people. During the Spring Festival, families get together and also pay New Year greetings to relatives and friends. From the perspective of strong connection and weak connection, "Spring Festival Greeting Networks" reflects the unique manifestation of social networks in China and has been used as a common way of measuring social networks in recent years [68,69]. In view of this, the number of relatives and friends who paid New Year greetings by calling or visiting in the Spring Festival of 2018 was selected to measure the scale of residents' social networks [34]. Secondly, since the samples selected in this study were rural residents, most of whom were engaged in agricultural activities or types of work other than as teachers, doctors, civil servants, and other public servants in public institutions, the number of public servants among residents' relatives and friends was selected to measure the heterogeneity of their social networks. In addition, cash gifts for marriage and funerals are an important embodiment of the substance transfer function of social networks in China. Therefore, the frequency of gift expenditure by households in 2018 was used to measure the substance transfer function of residents' social networks. Finally, the information transfer function was measured via a Likert scale, with 1 representing complete disagreement and 5 representing complete agreement with the statement "You often get disaster-related information from friends and relatives".

As distinct from flat social networks, another core variable that this study focused on was the degree of trust residents have in community management organizations. In China, the village is the most basic unit of rural society and provides the long-term community in which villagers live and work. As an autonomous form of organization at the grass-roots level in China, villagers' autonomous committees are responsible for the management of villagers and village-level affairs. Therefore, this study mainly investigated villagers' trust in their village committee. Referring to research on the definition and measurement of trust by McAllister [70], Luo et al. [71], Lee et al. [72], Ahsan and Dewan [73], Han et al. [74] and Peng, Tan, Lin, and Xu [18], this study designed entries to measure residents' trust in community management organizations in terms of three dimensions: cognitive trust, emotional trust, and organizational trust. Relating to these, the preconditions for high cognitive trust are reliable performance and excellent technical ability [75,76], which can encourage residents to establish positive cooperative relations with the community and be willing to seek information and help from community management organizations. High-caliber emotional trust is formed from harmonious community relations and friendly interpersonal communication; it reflects the emotional bond between community members and can promote mutual understanding and inclusiveness between residents and community management organizations. Organizational trust is a comprehensive concept that indicates residents' overall degree of trust in the community management system. It is worth noting that village committees belong to the most basic level of Chinese Government management organizations, so the trust levels of residents in the community management system was evaluated in terms of their degree of trust in the overall governmental system. The specific measures of cognitive trust, emotional trust, and organizational trust are shown in Table 3.

Table 3. Measurement of residents' degree of trust in community management organizations.

Entry Code	Dimension	Item [a]	Mean	SD [b]
CT1	Cognitive trust	In the face of future disasters, the community management organization has taken active preparedness measures.	3.92	1.00
CT2		If a disaster occurs, the community management organization will provide information on what to do.	4.12	0.94
AT1	Emotional trust	You are proud to live in this community.	3.82	1.10
AT2		Living in this village will give you more satisfaction than living anywhere else.	4.11	0.92
OT1	Organizational trust	In general, you have faith in government organizations.	4.46	0.84
OT2		People in the community have faith in the decisions of the government.	4.28	0.88

Note: [a] The Likert scale was used for all entries, with 1 representing complete disagreement and 5 representing complete agreement; [b] SD = standard deviation.

The specific measurement process for trust variables was the same as for the measurement of disaster-risk perception, and therefore will not be repeated here. In the reliability test, Cronbach α values corresponding to cognitive trust, emotional trust, organizational trust, and overall trust levels were all greater than 0.60 (0.71, 0.69, 0.66, and 0.70, respectively), indicating that the entries designed by this paper were internally consistent. In factor analysis, the Kaiser–Meyer–Olkin value corresponding to factor analysis was 0.65, the P value of the Bartlett test for sphericity was 0.000 (less than 0.001), and the cumulative variance contribution rate of the three dimensions was 77.09%, which indicated that the results of the factor analysis were reasonable (see Table 4 for details).

(3) Control variables

Referring to previous studies on the options of control variables (Salvati, Bianchi, Fiorucci, Giostrella, Marchesini, and Guzzetti [15], Devilliers and Maharaj [29], Xu, Qing, Deng, Yong, and Ma [33], Armas [77], Kellens et al. [78]), this paper selected the following as control variables that may correlate with residents' disaster-risk perception: individual characteristics, family characteristics, community characteristics, and characteristics of disaster experience. Specifically, individual characteristics were represented by gender, age, marital status, duration of residence, and education; family characteristics were described by family population, home address, and annual household income; community characteristics were described in terms of the status of disaster prevention and control in the community and the number of people threatened by disasters in the community;

and, disaster experience characteristics were reflected by the number of disasters and the severity of disasters experienced. The definitions of the model variables and the data descriptions are provided in Table 5.

Table 4. The component matrixes of each trust component after rotation.

Items	Component		
	Cognitive Trust	Emotional Trust	Organizational Trust
CT1	0.87	0.10	0.10
CT2	0.84	0.11	0.20
AT1	0.14	0.87	0.05
AT2	0.06	0.87	0.14
OT1	0.03	0.13	0.90
OT2	0.36	0.07	0.77
Eigenvalue	1.62	1.54	1.47
Explained variance	26.95%	25.67%	24.47%
Cumulative variance	26.95%	52.62%	77.09%
Cronbach α	0.71	0.69	0.66

Table 5. Definition of model variables and data description ($n = 327$).

Category		Variable	Definition and Measure	Mean	Standard Deviation
Dependent variables	Disaster-risk perceptions	Probability	Scores for perception of the possibility of disasters. [a]	49.81	19.63
		Threat	Scores for perception of the threat of disasters. [a]	60.56	19.18
		Self-efficacy	Scores for perception of their ability to take action to prevent disasters. [a]	64.36	21.73
		Response efficacy	Scores for perception of the effectiveness of response measures against disasters. [a]	77.94	16.75
		Comprehensive perception	Scores for comprehensive perception of disasters. [a]	63.7	9.62
Focal variables	Social networks	Network scale	The number of households of relatives and friends who visited or called during the Spring Festival of 2018 (households).	13.39	15.84
		Network heterogeneity	The number of relatives and friends working in public institutions (persons).	1.5	3
		Substance transfer function	The number of times of cash gifts given by households in 2018 (times).	18.78	17.28
		Information transfer function	You often get disaster-related information from friends and relatives. [b]	3.37	1.28
	Trust	Cognitive trust	The degree of cognitive trust in community management organizations. [a]	64.34	18.01
		Emotional trust	The degree of emotional trust in community management organizations. [a]	62.71	20.75
		Organizational trust	The degree of overall trust in the management system. [a]	73.32	18.53

Table 5. Cont.

Category	Variable		Definition and Measure	Mean	Standard Deviation
Control variables	Individual characteristics	Gender	Responder's gender (female = 1, male = 0).	0.46	0.5
		Age	Responder's age (years old).	53.41	13.5
		Marital status	Responder's marital status (married = 1, unmarried, widowed or divorced = 0).	0.87	0.35
		Duration of residence	Length of residence of responder (years).	42.63	25.54
		Education	Years of education (years).	6.29	3.7
	Family characteristics	Family population	Family population (persons).	4.13	1.82
		Home address	Is your home address within the disaster threat zone? (yes = 1, no = 0).	0.53	0.50
		Annual household income	Total annual cash income of household (yuan [c]). Households (yuan [c]).	66,185.17	72,280.03
	Community characteristics	Disaster prevention	The community has taken some measures to prevent/control disasters. [b]	3.89	1.08
		Number of people threatened by disasters	The number of people in the community threatened by disasters (persons).	212.65	247.65
	Characteristics of disaster experience	Number of times	The number of times of disaster experience (times).	8.8	12.04
		Severity	In general, how serious are the disasters you have experienced? (Likert scale, not very serious = 1, very serious = 5).	4.52	0.79

Note: [a] Centesimal system (0–100); [b] Likert scale with 1 representing complete disagreement and 5 representing complete agreement; [c] 1 USD = 7.09 yuan (at the time of the study).

2.3.2. Theoretical Analyses and Research Hypotheses

In terms of social network factors, different characteristics of residents' social networks may have distinct effects on their perceptions of disaster risks in each dimension. Social networks contain abundant material and information resources. Specifically, for elderly rural residents in mountainous areas, social networks may be an important way to obtain some material or information resources, but are also a crucial channel to obtain social support and security [79]. First, the scale and heterogeneity indicate the background of residents' social networks; the larger the scale and the stronger the heterogeneity, the more likely residents are to get material and emotional support from the networks. As a result, they may be "fearless", underestimating the possibility and threat of disasters and overestimating their perceptions of self-efficacy and response efficacy [74,80]. Secondly, although both substance and information transfer functions represent residents' use of social networks, substance transfer focuses on protection from risks, while information transfer focuses on the prediction of risks. Therefore, although theoretically the effect of the substance transfer function should be same as that of network scale and heterogeneity, the difference is that the more frequently residents transmit disaster-related information (especially information relating to the occurrence of and harm caused by disasters), the more likely they are to have enhanced perception of the possibility and threat of disasters, thereby weakening their self-efficacy and response efficacy evaluations [37,81].

In terms of trust factors, the degree of trust in community management organizations provided a comprehensive evaluation of the long-term performance of the management organizations by residents, concretely reflecting their reliability judgment of the community management organization's ability to cope with disaster risks. The higher the degree of trust, the more willing residents are to establish a positive cooperative relationship with the community and actively seek information and help from the community management organization [82,83]. At the same time, a high level of trust will form a strong emotional bond within the community, which can provide strong emotional support for residents and thus reduce their fear of disaster risks [84,85]. Therefore, in theory, a high level of trust may reduce residents' perceptions of the possibility and threat of disasters while increasing their perceptions of the self-efficacy and response efficacy [11,40,86].

According to existing literature conclusions and theoretical analyses, the following hypotheses were proposed for the relationship between rural residents' social networks, trust, and their disaster-risk perceptions:

Hypothesis 1 (H1). *There is a significant correlation between the social networks of rural residents in mountainous areas and their disaster-risk perceptions. Specifically:*

Hypothesis 1a (H1a). *The scale, heterogeneity, and substance transfer function of rural residents' social networks are significantly and negatively correlated with their possibility and threat perceptions of disaster risks, significantly and positively correlated with their self-efficacy and response efficacy, and significantly correlated with their comprehensive perceptions—with unclear effect.*

Hypothesis 1b (H1b). *The information transfer function of rural residents' social networks is significantly positively correlated with their possibility and threat perception of disaster risks, significantly and negatively correlated with their self-efficacy and response efficacy, and significantly correlated with the comprehensive perception—with unclear effect.*

Hypothesis 2 (H2). *There is a significant correlation between rural residents' trust in community management organizations and their perception of disaster risks. Specifically, cognitive trust, emotional trust, and organizational trust are significantly and negatively correlated with their possibility and threat perceptions of disaster risks, significantly and positively correlated with their self-efficacy and response efficacy, and significantly correlated with their comprehensive perception—with unclear effect.*

2.3.3. The Models

The dependent variables in this study were rural residents' perception of disaster risks. According to the data types and distribution characteristics of the dependent variables, this study used the Ordinary Least Squares (OLS) regression to control the characteristics of the individual, family, and community, and then gradually added social networks and trust variables to explore their correlations with residents' perceptions of disaster risks. The model was constructed according to Equation (3):

$$Y_i = \beta_{0i} + \beta_{1i} \times Control_i + \beta_{2i} \times social\ network_i + \beta_{3i} \times trust_i + \varepsilon_i \quad (3)$$

where Y_i refers to the model-dependent variables, specifically including the five indicators of possibility, threat, self-efficacy, response efficacy, and comprehensive perception; $Control_i$ represents the model control variables, including individual characteristics, family characteristics, community characteristics, and characteristics of disaster experience; $social\ network_i$ represents the model focal variables relating to social network indicators; and $trust_i$ represents the model focal variables relating to trust in community management organisations. In addition, β_{0i}, β_{1i}, β_{2i}, and β_{3i} are the parameters of the model to be estimated, and ε_i represents model residuals. Analysis of the models in this study was carried out by using Stata 13.0.

3. Results
3.1. Descriptive Statistics of the Variables

As shown in Table 5, in terms of the dependent variable of residents' perceptions of disaster risks, the average scores of the four dimensions of possibility, threat, self-efficacy, and response efficacy, as well as comprehensive perception, were 49.81, 60.56, 64.36, 77.94, and 63.70, respectively. Considering these findings as well as the means of the entries for each dimension of disaster-risk perception in Table 1 (the means of the entries for the five dimensions were 3.02, 3.48, 3.82, 4.32, and 3.66, respectively), and taking the mean score of comprehensive perception as the dividing line, the average perception score of the possibility and threat of disaster risks was lower, while the average perception scores of self-efficacy and response efficacy was higher. The reason for this may be that higher evaluations of their self-efficacy and response efficacy reduced residents' perceptions of the possibility and threat of disaster risk.

In terms of social network variables, the average network scale was 13.39 households; however, the mean value of network heterogeneity was only 1.5 persons. Additionally, the mean of the substance transfer function of social networks was 18.78 times. The mean of the information transfer function of social networks was 3.37, indicating that the frequency of information transfer of social networks was above the intermediate level with a score of 3. Regarding trust variables, the average score of cognitive trust, emotional trust, and organizational trust was 64.63, 62.71, and 73.32, respectively. Considering these findings in combination with the means of entries for each trust variable dimension in Table 3 (the means of the entries for the three aspects were 4.02, 3.97, and 4.37, respectively) indicated that the degree of trust in the management organization was at a higher level.

In terms of individual characteristics, the rural residents were mainly middle-aged, married, and male. Specifically, the average age of the residents was 53.41 years old, 87% were married and 54% were male. In addition, the average education level was 6.29 years and the average duration of residence in the current family was 42.63 years. In terms of family characteristics, 53% of the 327 rural residents believed that their families were in disaster-threatened areas, the average population of the sample families was 4.13, and the average annual household income was 66,185.17 yuan. The annual household income fluctuated greatly, indicating that there were considerable differences among sampled individuals. In terms of community characteristics, the main terrain of all 16 sample villages was mountainous land, and the mean disaster prevention value in communities was 3.89, indicating that most residents believed that some disaster prevention measures had been taken in the community. The average number of people threatened by disasters in communities was 212.65 persons. In terms of the disaster experience of the sampled residents, the average number of disasters experienced by residents was 8.80, but there was large fluctuation in this value. The mean value of the severity evaluation of the disasters experienced was 4.52, indicating that most residents believed that the disasters they had experienced were relatively serious.

3.2. Model Results

First, the Spearman rank correlation coefficient was used to test whether there was multiple collinearity between focal variables of the model (Table 6). The results showed that the correlation coefficients between focal variables were far less than 0.8, indicating that there was no serious multicollinearity between focal variables. Secondly, corresponding to the five dimensions of disaster-risk perception—including the possibility, threat, self-efficacy, response efficacy, and comprehensive perception—and considering the role of focal variables in the model, this study constructed 15 multiple linear regression models by gradually adding in the social network and trust variables (Tables 7–9). Relating to the dependent-variable indicators, the first model was the estimated result that only incorporated control variables, the second model estimated the result from addition of social network variables to the first model, and the third model estimated the result from addition of trust variables to the second model.

Table 6. Spearman rank correlation coefficient matrix of focal and control variables in the models.

Variable	1	2	3	4	5	6	7	8	9	10	11	12	13	14	15	16	17	18	19
1	1.000																		
2	0.000	1.000																	
3	0.000	0.000	1.000																
4	0.079	0.058	−0.035	1.000															
5	0.116 **	0.086	−0.139 **	0.346 ***	1.000														
6	0.006	−0.022	0.068	0.018	0.036	1.000													
7	−0.026	0.071	0.039	0.192 ***	0.164 ***	0.042	1.000												
8	−0.047	−0.063	−0.063	0.164 ***	−0.099 *	0.068	−0.015	1.000											
9	−0.132 **	0.095 *	0.197 ***	−0.066	−0.091	0.037	−0.043	−0.208 ***	1.000										
10	−0.053	0.102 *	0.132 **	−0.009	−0.033	0.109 **	0.061	−0.169 ***	0.405 ***	1.000									
11	0.043	0.051	−0.102 *	0.232 ***	0.327 ***	−0.103 *	0.108 *	−0.135 **	−0.494 ***	−0.210 ***	1.000								
12	0.064	−0.034	−0.008	0.130 *	0.099 *	0.027	0.107 *	0.104 *	0.067	−0.014	0.037	1.000							
13	−0.085	−0.236 ***	−0.065	0.132 **	0.118 **	0.027	−0.059	0.156 ***	−0.035	0.046	−0.087	−0.126 **	1.000						
14	0.119 ***	−0.104 *	−0.077	0.192 ***	0.054	0.080	0.192 ***	0.084	−0.314 ***	−0.180 ***	0.187 ***	0.249 ***	−0.026	1.000					
15	0.156 ***	0.029	0.022	0.262 ***	0.245 ***	0.039	−0.094 *	−0.059	−0.140 **	−0.141 **	0.246 **	0.051	−0.179 ***	0.314 ***	1.000				
16	0.517 ***	0.071	0.089	0.020	0.080	−0.052	0.046	−0.028	−0.039	−0.035	0.086	0.017	−0.036	0.021	0.103 *	1.000			
17	−0.069	−0.029	−0.137 **	0.012	0.124 **	0.060	0.118 **	−0.025	0.056	−0.033	0.082	0.013	0.051	0.036	0.094 *	−0.119 **	1.000		
18	−0.055	−0.012	0.003	0.073	−0.064	0.160 ***	0.046	0.031	0.006	0.009	−0.035	−0.017	0.062	0.033	0.094 *	−0.038	0.149 ***	1.000	
19	−0.015	−0.098 **	0.027	0.071	0.045	0.057	−0.032	−0.005	0.142 **	0.109 **	−0.107 *	0.060	0.196 ***	0.015	0.177 ***	−0.114 **	0.151 ***	0.124 **	1.000

Note: *** $p < 0.01$, ** $p < 0.05$, * $p < 0.1$. 1—cognitive trust, 2—emotional trust, 3—organizational trust, 4—network scale, 5—network heterogeneity, 6—substance transfer function of social networks, 7—information transfer function of social networks, 8—gender, 9—age, 10—duration of residence, 11—education, 12—marital status, 13—home address, 14—family population, 15—annual household income, 16—disaster prevention in the community, 17—number of people threatened by disasters in the community, 18—severity of disasters experienced by the respondent, 19—number of times of disasters experienced by the respondent.

Table 7. Estimation results of the impact of social networks and trust on rural residents' possibility and threat perceptions of disaster risks in a multi-disaster environment (standardization coefficient).

Variables	Possibility			Threat		
	Model 1	Model 2	Model 3	Model 4	Model 5	Model 6
Gender	−0.092 (−1.557)	−0.094 (−1.587)	−0.103 * (−1.740)	−0.099 * (−1.716)	−0.099 * (−1.682)	−0.102 * (−1.722)
Age	0.048 (0.651)	0.047 (0.646)	0.035 (0.469)	−0.192 *** (−2.685)	−0.194 *** (−2.700)	−0.192 ** (−2.585)
Duration of residence	−0.024 (−0.399)	−0.046 (−0.759)	−0.057 (−0.942)	0.029 (0.490)	0.038 (0.628)	0.041 (0.670)
Education	−0.062 (−0.921)	−0.063 (−0.911)	−0.078 (−1.113)	−0.199 *** (−3.016)	−0.213 *** (−3.090)	−0.215 *** (−3.080)
Marital status	−0.024 (−0.423)	−0.034 (−0.582)	−0.024 (−0.409)	0.002 (0.031)	0.002 (0.032)	0.003 (0.055)
Home address	0.163 *** (2.810)	0.167 *** (2.879)	0.197 *** (3.321)	0.094 (1.639)	0.093 (1.628)	0.092 (1.549)
Family population	0.009 (0.140)	−0.018 (−0.292)	−0.007 (−0.111)	0.018 (0.288)	0.032 (0.510)	0.032 (0.508)
Annual household income	−0.141 ** (−2.287)	−0.158 ** (−2.524)	−0.153 ** (−2.461)	−0.079 (−1.303)	−0.079 (−1.275)	−0.074 (−1.194)
Disaster prevention in the community	−0.088 (−1.580)	−0.075 (−1.348)	−0.072 (−1.102)	−0.126 ** (−2.297)	−0.130 ** (−2.356)	−0.113 * (−1.732)
Number of people threatened by disasters in the community	0.024 (0.435)	0.020 (0.360)	0.018 (0.310)	0.051 (0.919)	0.048 (0.856)	0.042 (0.739)
Severity of disasters experienced	0.082 (1.494)	0.055 (0.971)	0.052 (0.925)	0.133 ** (2.457)	0.149 *** (2.687)	0.148 *** (2.642)
Number of times of disasters experienced	0.000 (0.000)	0.006 (0.103)	0.017 (0.285)	−0.198 *** (−3.445)	−0.199 *** (−3.415)	−0.195 *** (−3.324)
Network scale		0.030 (0.489)	0.026 (0.430)		−0.037 (−0.609)	−0.037 (−0.614)
Network heterogeneity		−0.002 (−0.035)	−0.013 (−0.212)		0.047 (0.764)	0.040 (0.639)
Substance transfer function		0.106 * (1.905)	0.111 ** (2.012)		−0.071 (−1.295)	−0.066 (−1.204)
Information transfer function		0.093 (1.637)	0.086 (1.519)		−0.004 (−0.079)	−0.002 (−0.031)
Cognitive trust			−0.020 (−0.302)			−0.025 (−0.383)
Emotional trust			0.149 *** (2.646)			0.013 (0.227)
Organizational trust			−0.038 (−0.667)			−0.049 (−0.863)
N	327	327	327	327	327	327
F	2.654 ***	2.439 ***	2.495 ***	3.700 ***	2.905 ***	2.480 ***
R^2	0.092	0.112	0.134	0.124	0.130	0.133
Adjusted R^2	0.057	0.066	0.080	0.090	0.086	0.079

Note: The values in parentheses indicate the corresponding T values; *** indicates significant at the 1% level, ** indicates significant at the 5% level, and * indicates significant at the 10% level.

Table 8. Estimation results of the impact of social networks and trust on rural residents' self-efficacy and response efficacy of disaster risks in a multi-disaster environment (standardization coefficient).

Variables	Self-Efficacy			Response Efficacy		
	Model 7	Model 8	Model 9	Model 10	Model 11	Model 12
Gender	−0.104 * (−1.836)	−0.099 * (−1.742)	−0.091 (−1.648)	−0.036 (−0.604)	−0.035 (−0.591)	−0.031 (−0.536)
Age	−0.085 (−1.206)	−0.086 (−1.226)	−0.072 (−1.035)	0.042 (0.576)	0.040 (0.554)	0.001 (0.018)
Duration of residence	0.048 (0.835)	0.030 (0.522)	−0.004 (−0.076)	−0.049 (−0.815)	−0.060 (−0.999)	−0.081 (−1.356)
Education	0.235 *** (3.649)	0.243 *** (3.648)	0.255 *** (3.886)	0.075 (1.121)	0.088 (1.275)	0.079 (1.155)
Marital status	0.099 * (1.786)	0.091 (1.639)	0.094 * (1.731)	0.072 (1.249)	0.069 (1.191)	0.074 (1.311)
Home address	0.002 (0.034)	0.005 (0.090)	0.060 (1.071)	0.020 (0.335)	0.017 (0.296)	0.047 (0.812)
Family population	0.057 (0.955)	0.021 (0.344)	0.027 (0.464)	0.015 (0.235)	−0.016 (−0.261)	−0.003 (−0.055)
Annual household income	0.076 (1.284)	0.063 (1.055)	0.049 (0.845)	−0.017 (−0.280)	−0.020 (−0.327)	−0.037 (−0.603)
Disaster prevention in the community	0.135 ** (2.512)	0.152 *** (2.829)	0.028 (0.461)	0.013 (0.224)	0.036 (0.639)	−0.015 (−0.226)
Number of people threatened by disasters in the community	−0.009 (−0.174)	−0.002 (−0.034)	0.009 (0.161)	−0.063 (−1.110)	−0.051 (−0.913)	−0.020 (−0.366)
Severity of disasters experienced	0.038 (0.724)	0.004 (0.076)	0.012 (0.231)	0.258 *** (4.671)	0.232 *** (4.142)	0.236 *** (4.310)
Number of times of disasters experienced	−0.003 (−0.060)	0.003 (0.062)	0.000 (0.003)	0.090 (1.532)	0.109 * (1.853)	0.1000 * (1.738)
Network scale		0.088 (1.521)	0.081 (1.432)		0.021 (0.340)	0.021 (0.360)
Network heterogeneity		−0.082 (−1.379)	−0.089 (−1.534)		−0.110 * (−1.784)	−0.076 (−1.259)
Substance transfer function		0.077 (1.440)	0.070 (1.347)		−0.020 (−0.364)	−0.039 (−0.718)
Information transfer function		0.096 * (1.755)	0.082 (1.531)		0.161 *** (2.831)	0.139 ** (2.495)
Cognitive trust			0.200 *** (3.302)			0.041 (0.653)
Emotional trust			0.172 *** (3.251)			0.058 (1.058)
Organizational trust			0.068 (1.293)			0.234 *** (4.241)
N	327	327	327	327	327	327
F	4.969 ***	4.302 ***	4.982 ***	2.507 ***	2.578 ***	3.278 ***
R^2	0.160	0.182	0.236	0.087	0.117	0.169
Adjusted R^2	0.127	0.139	0.188	0.053	0.072	0.117

Note: The values in parentheses indicate the corresponding T values; *** indicates significant at the 1% level, ** indicates significant at the 5% level, and * indicates significant at the 10% level.

Table 9. Estimation results of the impact of social networks and trust on rural residents' comprehensive perceptions for disaster risks in a multi-disaster environment (standardization coefficient).

Variables	Comprehensive Perception		
	Model 13	Model 14	Model 15
Gender	−0.165 *** (−2.840)	−0.163 *** (−2.813)	−0.163 *** (−2.875)
Age	−0.086 (−1.192)	−0.088 (−1.244)	−0.106 (−1.485)
Duration of residence	0.002 (0.034)	−0.021 (−0.348)	−0.054 (−0.923)
Education	0.043 (0.650)	0.047 (0.687)	0.04 (0.591)
Marital status	0.077 (1.355)	0.066 (1.172)	0.076 (1.379)
Home address	0.137 ** (2.385)	0.139 ** (2.453)	0.198 *** (3.482)
Family population	0.05 (0.819)	0.008 (0.125)	0.024 (0.393)
Annual household income	−0.076 (−1.246)	−0.093 (−1.519)	−0.104 * (−1.743)
Disaster prevention in the community	−0.023 (−0.422)	0.002 (0.035)	−0.08 (−1.272)
Number of people threatened by disasters in the community	−0.001 (−0.015)	0.005 (0.097)	0.022 (0.410)
Severity of disasters experienced	0.25 *** (4.605)	0.212 *** (3.862)	0.216 *** (4.034)
Number of times of disasters experienced	−0.046 (−0.790)	−0.03 (−0.518)	−0.029 (−0.511)
Network scale		0.057 (0.955)	0.051 (0.879)
Network heterogeneity		−0.078 (−1.302)	−0.075 (−1.260)
Substance transfer function		0.054 (0.994)	0.046 (0.866)
Information transfer function		0.178 *** (3.185)	0.157 *** (2.872)
Cognitive trust			0.107 * (1.723)
Emotional trust			0.204 *** (3.772)
Organizational trust			0.112 ** (2.067)
N	327	327	327
F	3.394 ***	3.428 ***	4.100 ***
R^2	0.115	0.150	0.202
Adjusted R^2	0.081	0.106	0.153

Note: The values in parentheses indicate the corresponding T values; *** indicates significant at the 1% level, ** indicates significant at the 5% level, and * indicates significant at the 10% level.

The F test results (Tables 7–9) showed that the overall significance of all models was below the 1%, meaning that at least one of the focal variables was significantly correlated with the dependent variables. Comparison of the adjusted R^2 values of the three models in each dependent variable dimension revealed that, with the exception of the adjusted R^2 value of the threat perception which decreased with the addition of focal variables, the adjusted R^2 values of the remaining four dependent variables all significantly increased with the addition of the social network and trust variables. Specifically, for models 1–15, sequentially, the goodness of fit for the probability perception was 5.7%, 6.6%, and 8.0%, respectively; the goodness of fit for the threat perception was 9.0%, 8.6%, and 7.9%, respectively; the goodness of fit for self-efficacy was 12.7%, 13.9%, and 18.8%, respectively; the goodness of fit for response efficacy was 5.3%, 7.2%, and 11.7% respectively; and, the goodness of fit for comprehensive perception was 8.1%, 10.6%, and 15.3%, respectively. Due to the goodness of fit of models 3, 4, 9, 12, and 15, this study focused on the estimation results of these five models and combined these with other models of each dependent variable for the subsequent results analysis.

It can be seen from the estimated results of model 3 (Table 7) that residents' perceptions of the possibility of disaster risks were significantly and positively correlated with the information transfer function of residents' social networks ($p < 0.05$) and emotional trust in the community management organization ($p < 0.01$). Specifically speaking, when other conditions remained unchanged, for every one unit increase in the information transfer function of residents' social networks, their perceptions of the probability of disaster risks increased by 0.111 units, on average; and, for every one unit increase in the emotional trust in the community management organization, their perceptions of the probability of disaster risks increased by 0.149 units, on average. In addition, control variables of gender ($p < 0.1$) and annual household income ($p < 0.01$) both had significant negative impacts on residents' possibility perceptions of disaster risk, while the home address ($p < 0.01$) had a significant and positive impact on residents' perceptions of the possibility of disaster risk. In other words, male residents with low annual household income and whose home addresses are threatened by disasters tended to think that disasters were more likely to occur.

Regarding residents' perceptions of the threat of disaster risks, after adding social network and trust variables on the basis of model 4, which contained only control variables, the goodness of fit of model 6 was reduced; this may have been caused by the insignificant effects of the two focal variables on the threat perception of disaster risk. As the estimation results of model 4 had good goodness of fit for the threat-perception models shown (Table 7), gender ($p < 0.1$), age ($p < 0.01$), education ($p < 0.01$), the number of disasters experienced, and disaster prevention in their communities ($p < 0.05$) were significantly and negatively correlated with the perceived threat of disaster risks. However, the severity of the disasters experienced by the resident ($p < 0.05$) was significantly positively correlated with the perceived threat of disaster risk. The estimation results of model 5 and model 6 (Table 7) revealed the same significant variables as for model 4, but several variables (age, disaster prevention in communities, and severity of experienced disasters) were distinguishing at significant levels. Therefore, on the basis of the estimation results of these three models, it was concluded that male residents who were younger, less educated, and less prepared for disasters in their communities, and had experienced fewer disasters but more severe ones, had higher perceived threat of disaster risk.

In terms of residents' perceptions of self-efficacy relating to disaster risks, it can be seen from the estimated results of model 9 (Table 8) that cognitive trust ($p < 0.01$) and emotional trust ($p < 0.01$) were significantly and positively correlated with residents' perceptions of self-efficacy relating to disaster risks, while social networks had no significant effect on their self-efficacy perceptions. To be specific, when other conditions remained unchanged, for every one unit increase in cognitive trust in the community management organization, residents' perceptions of self-efficacy relating to disaster risks increased by 0.200 units, on average; and, for every one unit increase in emotional trust in the community management organization, their perceptions of self-efficacy relating to disaster risks increased by 0.172 units, on average. It is also worth noting that, according to the estimated results of model 8 (Table 8), the substance transfer function of residents' social networks was significantly positively correlated with their self-efficacy perceptions (at the 0.1 level). However, this feature was no longer significant after the inclusion of trust variables, which may have been caused by the insufficient explanatory power of the substance transfer function of the social network compared to the impact of trust variables on the self-efficacy of residents. In addition, the control variables of education ($p < 0.01$) and marital status ($p < 0.1$) both had significant and negative impacts on residents' self-efficacy perceptions relating to disaster risks. In other words, married residents who were more educated tended to think that they were better able to take action to prevent disasters.

In terms of residents' perceptions of the response efficacy relating to disaster risks, according to the estimated results of model 12 (Table 8), the substance transfer function of residents' social networks ($p < 0.05$) and organizational trust ($p < 0.01$) were both significantly and positively correlated with the response efficacy for disaster risks. Specifically speaking, when other conditions remained unchanged, for every one unit increase in the substance transfer function of residents' social networks, their perceptions of response efficacy of disaster risks increased by 0.139 units, on average; and, for every one unit increase in organizational trust in the community management organization, their perceptions of response efficacy relating to disaster risks increased by 0.234 units, on average. In addition, the control variables of the severity of experienced disasters ($p < 0.01$) and the number of experienced disasters ($p < 0.01$) both had significant positive impacts on residents' perceptions of response efficacy relating to disaster risks. In other words, the more severe and frequent disasters experienced by residents, the stronger their perceptions of response efficacy relating to disaster risks.

In terms of residents' comprehensive perceptions of disaster risks, according to the estimated results of model 15 (Table 9), the substance transfer function of residents' social networks ($p < 0.01$), cognitive trust ($p < 0.1$), emotional trust ($p < 0.01$), and organizational trust ($p < 0.01$) were significantly positively correlated with their comprehensive perceptions of disaster risks. Specifically, when other conditions remained unchanged, for every one unit increase in the substance transfer function of residents' social networks, their comprehensive perceptions of disaster risks increased by 0.157 units, on average; for every one unit increase in cognitive trust, residents' comprehensive perceptions of disaster risks increased by 0.107 units, on average; for every one unit increase in emotional trust, residents' comprehensive perceptions of disaster risks increased by 0.204 units, on average; and, for every one unit increase in organizational trust, residents' comprehensive perceptions of disaster risks increased by 0.112 units, on average. Additionally, control variables of the home address ($p < 0.01$) and the severity of experienced disasters ($p < 0.01$) had significant positive impacts on residents' comprehensive perceptions of disaster risks, while gender ($p < 0.01$) and annual household income ($p < 0.1$) were significantly negatively correlated with their comprehensive perceptions of disaster risks. In other words, male residents with low annual household income and addresses threatened by disasters, who had experienced more severe disasters, had a higher comprehensive perception of disaster risks.

Combining the findings of all the above models revealed the following. First, the background characteristics of residents' social networks were not significantly correlated with their disaster-risk perceptions, while the substance and information carrier function of social networks were significantly correlated with some dimensions of disaster-risk perceptions. This suggested that social network variables affecting residents' disaster-risk perception did not relate to background characteristics but to the use of social networks. Second, compared with social network variables, trust variables were more closely related to the perceived level of disaster risks, which was especially reflected in the correlation with self-efficacy, response efficacy, and comprehensive perception of disaster risks. More specifically, the estimated results of self-efficacy (model 9) showed that trust variables were significantly correlated with self-efficacy perception, while social network variables were not; the estimated results of response efficacy (models 11 and 12) showed that after the addition of trust variables, the effect of substance transfer function on the response efficacy perception decreased in both intensity and significance, and the effect was much smaller than that of the organizational trust variable; the estimated results of comprehensive perception (model 15) showed that the three dimensions of trust variables were significantly correlated with comprehensive perception, while only the social network substance transfer function was significantly correlated with comprehensive perception. The reason for these findings may be due to the response measures of sampled residents to disasters being more concentrated at the public level (such as setting disaster warning boards, planning evacuation routes, etc.), and less at the individual or family level. In this context of public disaster prevention, the degree of trust in management organizations will undoubtedly be more closely related to the level of disaster-risk perceptions. It was worth noting that all of the significant social network variables and trust variables had positive effects on the corresponding dimensions of disaster-risk perceptions, which indicated that trust relating to both the flat social network and pyramidal channels positively affected residents' perceived levels of disaster risks.

4. Discussion

Compared with existing literature, this study made the following marginal contributions. First, previous studies mainly focused on residents' risk perceptions for single types of disasters, such as earthquakes, floods, and landslides, whereas this study took rural residents threatened by multiple disasters as the research object and measured their perception levels of multiple disaster risks. Second, in existing studies, the measurement of residents' disaster-risk perceptions mainly considered their understanding and feelings relating to the disaster event itself. This study attempted to evaluate residents' generalized disaster-risk perception levels from two aspects: their perceptions of the disaster-risk event itself and the degree of mitigation that could be achieved. Third, whereas previous studies did not focus strongly on the impact of social network factors on residents' perceptions of disaster risks, this study quantitatively explored the correlation between social network factors and residents' perceptions of disaster risks through the description of background characteristics and carrier characteristics of social networks. Fourth, as distinct from flat social networks, this paper incorporated pyramidal trust channels and empirically explored the correlation between these and residents' disaster-risk perceptions, as well as further analyzing the different impacts of social network and pyramidal trust factors on residents' perceptions of disaster risks.

Individual perception of disaster risks is not only the product of individual factors, but also the product of interpersonal and social interactions. In partial support of research hypotheses H1a and H1b, this study found that the information transfer function of social networks was significantly positively correlated with residents' perceptions of the possibility of disaster risks, and the substance transfer function had significant positive effect on their response efficacy and comprehensive perceptions of disaster risks. These results indicated that the more frequently residents transmitted disaster-related information, especially information relating to the occurrence of and harm caused by disasters, the more their perceptions of the possibility of disaster risks would be enhanced; meanwhile, the substance transfer function of social networks, as an important embodiment of residents' social support, could enable residents to get material support and security, thus affecting their perceptions of response efficacy. The above results of this paper were consistent with the findings of Iuliana et al. [87], Wu and Li [81] and Jones, Faas, Murphy, Tobin, and Mccarty [37]. For example, Iuliana, ArmaşEugen, and Avram [87] found that the material support residents received could enhance their safety perception levels relating to response measures; Jones, Faas, Murphy, Tobin, and Mccarty [37] found that the more frequent communication among residents, the higher their perception of the possibility of disaster risk. However, the findings of this paper were inconsistent with the findings of Grayscholz et al. [88], in which the background characteristics of social networks (network scale and network heterogeneity) were not significantly correlated with residents' perceived levels of disaster risks. The reason for this may be that, even though residents had good social network background characteristics, they did not make much use of the corresponding functions of social networks, which weakened the effect of social networks on their perceptions of disaster risks. Furthermore, the background characteristics of social networks represented the potential resources contained in social networks. The carrier characteristics of social networks reflected the mobilized resources. This also suggested that it is not the amount of social relationship resources you have, but the amount of social relationship resources you use that is the key to affect the residents' perceptions of disaster risks. To sum up, as the carrier of some social resources transmission, social networks can enable residents to obtain practical social securities through its specific functional characteristics, such as information transfer and material support, thus effectively affecting residents' disaster-risk perceptions. This finding indicates that social networks play an important role in disaster-risk management, which should be more noted.

The current disaster-prevention system in China is mainly community-based disaster prevention [89,90]. In this context, residents' trust in community management organizations greatly affects their perceptions of disaster risks. In partial support of research hypothesis H2, this study found that cognitive trust and emotional trust had significant positive effects on self-efficacy and comprehensive perceptions of disaster risks, while organizational trust was significantly positively correlated with response efficacy and comprehensive perceptions of disaster risks. The above results of this study were consistent with the findings of ter Huurne and Gutteling [91], Peng, Tan, Lin, and Xu [18] and Han, Wang, and Cui [40], who found that residents' trust in the public sector was significantly correlated with their perceptions of the controllability of disaster risks. However, inconsistent with research hypothesis H2 and the findings of Fátima and Bernardo [92] and Grayscholz, Haney, and Macquarrie [88], regression estimation results of this study showed that emotional trust was positively correlated with residents' perceptions of the possibility of disaster risks. This discrepancy in findings may be due to the following reasons. First, emotional trust reflects harmonious community relations and friendly interpersonal communication. The higher the emotional trust, the more frequent the communication between residents will be and the easier it will be to obtain disaster-related information, thus leading to increased perceptions of the possibility of disaster risks. Secondly, the residents in this study were more vulnerable to disasters (the average number of disasters experienced by the sample was 8.80 times). Based on this experience, high emotional trust may lead residents to fear that sudden disasters will harm their cherished communities, thus enhancing their perceptions of the possibility of disaster risks. In addition, it is worth noting that, different to the findings of Bronfman et al. [93] and Han, Xiaoli Lu, Elisa I. Hörhager, and Jubo Yan [74], the empirical results of this study showed that trust factors were not significantly correlated with perceptions of disaster risks. The possible reason is that, although residents believed that community management organizations would take various measures to reduce their losses caused by disasters, the disaster-prone environment still poses a threat to their lives and property. Compared with social network variables, trust variables were more closely related to the perceived level of disaster risk, which was especially reflected in its impact on self-efficacy, response efficacy, and comprehensive perception. This implies that residents paid more attention to the reliability of information and support—the characteristics of pyramid channels—rather than the repeated and uncertain information with high frequency. Furthermore, while information and substance provided by the social network was more convenient and quick, only when the social network implemented its carrier function, it showed close correlation with disaster-risk perception, which also reflected the actual rather than potential support was the vital factor correlating with disaster-risk perception.

In addition, this study found that residents' individual characteristics (gender, age, education, marital status), family characteristics (home address, annual household income), community characteristics (disaster prevention in the community), and characteristics of disaster experience (the number and severity of experienced disasters) were significantly correlated with different dimensions of the perception of disaster risks. This was consistent with some of the findings of Lindell and Hwang [94], Kellens, Zaalberg, Neutens, Vanneuville, and De Maeyer [78], Xu et al. [95], Ardaya et al. [96], and Tanner and Arvai [97]. For example, Kellens, Zaalberg, Neutens, Vanneuville, and De Maeyer [78] found that individuals' age, gender, and flood disaster experience significantly affected their perceptions of the threat of flood disaster risks; and Xu, Peng, Su, Liu, Wang, and Chen [95] found that the distance of respondents' houses from the disaster site and disaster experience were significantly correlated with their perceptions of the possibility of disaster risks. Similarly, the present study found that home addresses that were threatened by disasters significantly affected participants' perceptions of the possibility of disaster risks, and the age, gender, and disaster experience of participants were all significantly correlated with their perceived levels of the threat of disaster risks.

Although this study provides a useful exploration of the correlations between social networks, trust, and residents' disaster-risk perceptions, it had some deficiencies. In terms of measuring response efficacy, in consideration of the fact that this study dealt with multiple disasters, the response efficacy specifically referred to the degree to which evacuation could reduce the threat of disasters. However, residents' perceived effects of different disaster response behaviors might vary, and the perceived effects of other disaster prevention and mitigation measures (such as relocation, reinforcement of houses, etc.) were not considered in this study. In addition, the goal of disaster risk management is to prevent and avoid disasters. Due to the limited space, this study was not extended to include residents' behavioral responses to disasters. Therefore, future research could explore the differences in residents' perceptions of response efficacy of different disaster prevention and reduction measures, and the effects of social networks, trust, disaster-risk perceptions, and other factors on residents' behavioral responses to disasters could be further discussed.

5. Conclusions

Based on the empirical analysis and discussion above, this study formed the following main conclusions:

(1) In terms of the characteristics of rural residents' perceptions of disaster risks, compared with the disaster-risk comprehensive perception scores, participants had lower perception scores relating to possibility and threat and higher perception scores relating to self-efficacy and response efficacy.

(2) The variables of social network that affected residents' perceptions of disaster risks did not relate to their background characteristics of social networks, but to the use of their carrier characteristics. Specifically, the information transfer function of social networks had a significant positive effect on the perceived level of the possibility; the substance transfer function had a significant positive effect on the perceived level of the response efficacy and comprehensive perception, while the network scale and network heterogeneity had no significant impact on any dimension of disaster-risk perception.

(3) Different dimensions of trust had distinct effects on rural residents' disaster-risk perceptions. Specifically, emotional trust was significantly and positively correlated with the perception level of the possibility and self-efficacy of disaster risk, cognitive trust was significantly and positively correlated with self-efficacy and the comprehensive perception of disaster risk, and organizational trust was significantly and positively correlated with the perception of response efficacy and the comprehensive perception of disaster risk.

(4) Compared with social network variables, trust was more closely related to the perceived level of disaster risk, which was especially reflected in its impact on self-efficacy, response efficacy, and comprehensive perception.

It is only when residents are aware of the risks they face that they will respond accordingly. Based on the above analysis, in order to improve residents' perceptions of disaster risks and to strengthen the disaster-risk management ability of communities, this study has the following three suggestions. First, residents' communication groups or mutual aid groups could be established to strengthen daily contact between community residents and thereby improve residents' awareness of disaster risks; secondly, strengthening the training of community managers in disaster-related knowledge and organizing disaster prevention and avoidance activities in time to enhance residents' confidence in dealing with disaster risks could be an effective strategy; and thirdly, combining community disaster prevention with individual disaster prevention, through reasonable guidance, would take advantage of both pyramidal and flat channels in the construction of resilient disaster prevention systems. For example, on the basis of community disaster prevention, community managers can advocate mutual help to strengthen the substantive support between residents, and jointly improve the resilience of residents to confront disaster risks.

Author Contributions: Conceptualization, K.X., D.X., and S.L.; data curation, K.X. and S.G.; investigation, K.X. and Y.L.; funding acquisition, D.X.; supervision, S.L.; writing—original draft, K.X.; writing—review and editing, D.X. and S.L. All authors have read and agreed to the published version of the manuscript.

Funding: This research was funded by National Natural Science Foundation of China (Grant No. 41801221).

Institutional Review Board Statement: Not applicable.

Informed Consent Statement: Informed consent was obtained from all subjects involved in the study.

Acknowledgments: We sincerely thank our colleagues who provided some technical guidance for this research. The authors also extend special gratitude to the anonymous reviewers and editors for their comments in greatly improving the quality of this paper.

Conflicts of Interest: All authors declare no conflict of interest.

References

1. Steffen, W.; Sanderson, A.; Tyson, P.D.; Jaeger, J.; Matson, P.A.; Moore, B., III; Oldfleld, F.; Richardson, K.; Schellnhuber, H.J.; Turner, B.L., II; et al. *Global Change and the Earth System: A Planet under Pressure*; Springer: Cham, Switzerland, 2004; pp. 1–336.
2. Anzellini, V.; Desai, B.; Leduc, C. *Global Report on Internal Displacement (2020)*; The Internal Displacement Monitoring Centre: Geneva, Switzerland, 2020; p. 1.
3. Bevere, L.; Gloor, M.; Sobel, A. *Natural Catastrophes in Times of Economic Accumulation and Climate Change*; Swiss Re Institute: Zurich, Switzerland, 2020; p. 4.
4. Beniston, M. Climatic Change in Mountain Regions: A Review of Possible Impacts. *Clim. Chang.* **2003**, *59*, 5–31. [CrossRef]
5. Zimmermann, M.; Keiler, M. International Frameworks for Disaster Risk Reduction: Useful Guidance for Sustainable Mountain Development? *Mt. Res. Dev.* **2015**, *35*, 195–202. [CrossRef]
6. Fang, Y.P.; Jie, F.; Shen, M.Y.; Song, M.Q. Sensitivity of livelihood strategy to livelihood capital in mountain areas: Empirical analysis based on different settlements in the upper reaches of the Minjiang River, China. *Ecol. Indic.* **2014**, *38*, 225–235. [CrossRef]
7. Xu, D.; Zhang, J.; Golam, R.; Liu, S.; Xie, F.; Cao, M.; Liu, E. Household Livelihood Strategies and Dependence on Agriculture in the Mountainous Settlements in the Three Gorges Reservoir Area, China. *Sustainability* **2015**, *7*, 4850–4869. [CrossRef]
8. Zeng, X.; Guo, S.; Deng, X.; Wenfeng, Z.; Xu, D. Livelihood risk and adaptation strategies of farmers in earthquake hazard threatened areas: Evidence from sichuan province, China. *Int. J. Disaster Risk Reduct.* **2020**, *53*, 101971. [CrossRef]
9. Wenfeng, Z.; Guo, S.; Deng, X.; Xu, D.; Hazards, N. Livelihood resilience and strategies of rural residents of earthquake-threatened areas in Sichuan Province, China. *Nat. Hazards* **2021**, 1–21. [CrossRef]
10. Bureau, C.N.S. *China Statistical Yearbook in 2019*; China Statistical Press: Beijing, China, 2019. (In Chinese)
11. Siegrist, M.; Gutscher, H.; Earle, T.C. Perception of risk: The influence of general trust, and general confidence. *J. Risk Res.* **2005**, *8*, 145–156. [CrossRef]
12. Lindell, M.K.; Arlikatti, S.; Prater, C.S. Why People Do What They Do to Protect Against Earthquake Risk: Perceptions of Hazard Adjustment Attributes. *Risk Anal.* **2009**, *29*, 1072–1088. [CrossRef] [PubMed]
13. Damm, A.; Eberhard, K.; Sendzimir, J.; Patt, A. Perception of landslides risk and responsibility: A case study in eastern Styria, Austria. *Nat. Hazards* **2013**, *69*, 165–183. [CrossRef]
14. Morss, R.E.; Wilhelmi, O.V.; Downton, M.W.; Gruntfest, E. Flood Risk, Uncertainty, and Scientific Information for Decision Making: Lessons from an Interdisciplinary Project. *Bull. Am. Meteorol. Soc.* **2005**, *86*, 1593–1601. [CrossRef]
15. Salvati, P.; Bianchi, C.; Fiorucci, F.; Giostrella, P.; Marchesini, I.; Guzzetti, F. Perception of flood and landslide risk in Italy: A preliminary analysis. *Nat. Hazards Earth Syst. Sci.* **2014**, *14*, 2589–2603. [CrossRef]
16. Doyle, E.E.H.; John, M.C.; Potter, S.H.; Becker, J.S.; Johnston, D.M.; Lindell, M.K.; Sarbjit, J.; Fraser, S.A.; Coomer, M.A. Motivations to prepare after the 2013 Cook Strait Earthquake, N.Z. *Int. J. Disaster Risk Reduct.* **2018**, *31*, 637–649. [CrossRef]
17. Grothmann, T.; Reusswig, F. People at risk of flooding: Why some residents take precautionary action while others do not. *Nat. Hazards* **2006**, *38*, 101–120. [CrossRef]

18. Peng, L.; Tan, J.; Lin, L.; Xu, D. Understanding sustainable disaster mitigation of stakeholder engagement: Risk perception, trust in public institutions, and disaster insurance. *Sustain. Dev.* **2019**, *27*, 885–897. [CrossRef]
19. Miceli, R.; Sotgiu, I.; Settanni, M. Disaster preparedness and perception of flood risk: A study in an alpine valley in Italy. *J. Environ. Psychol.* **2008**, *28*, 164–173. [CrossRef]
20. Xu, D.; Peng, L.; Liu, S.; Wang, X. Influences of Risk Perception and Sense of Place on Landslide Disaster Preparedness in Southwestern China. *Int. J. Disaster Risk Sci.* **2018**, *9*, 167–180. [CrossRef]
21. Palm, R. Urban earthquake hazards: The impacts of culture on perceived risk and response in the USA and Japan. *Appl. Geogr.* **1998**, *18*, 35–46. [CrossRef]
22. Scolobig, A.; Marchi, B.D.; Borga, M. The missing link between flood risk awareness and preparedness: Findings from case studies in an Alpine Region. *Nat. Hazards* **2012**, *63*, 499–520. [CrossRef]
23. Xu, D.; Zhou, W.; Deng, X.; Ma, Z.; Yong, Z.; Qin, C. Information credibility, disaster risk perception and evacuation willingness of rural households in China. *Nat. Hazards* **2020**, *103*, 2865–2882. [CrossRef]
24. Mulilis, J.A.; Lippa, R. Behavioral Change in Earthquake Preparedness Due to Negative Threat Appeals: A Test of Protection Motivation Theory. *J. Appl. Soc. Psychol.* **1990**, *20*, 619–638. [CrossRef]
25. Zaalberg, R.; Midden, C.; Meijnders, A.; Mccalley, T. Prevention, Adaptation, and Threat Denial: Flooding Experiences in the Netherlands. *Risk Anal.* **2009**, *29*, 1759–1778. [CrossRef]
26. Mertens, K.; Jacobs, L.; Maes, J.; Poesen, J.; Kervyn, M.; Vranken, L. Disaster risk reduction among households exposed to landslide hazard: A crucial role for self-efficacy? *Land Use Policy* **2018**, *75*, 77–91. [CrossRef]
27. Wiegman, O.; Gutteling, J.M. Risk Appraisal and Risk Communication: Some Empirical Data from the Netherlands Reviewed. *Basic Appl. Soc. Psychol.* **1995**, *16*, 227–249. [CrossRef]
28. Bubeck, P.; Botzen, W.J.W.; Aerts, J.C.J.H. A Review of Risk Perceptions and Other Factors that Influence Flood Mitigation Behavior. *Risk Anal.* **2012**, *32*, 1481–1495. [CrossRef] [PubMed]
29. Devilliers, G.D.; Maharaj, R. Human perceptions and responses to floods with specific reference to the 1987 flood in the mdloti river near durban, south-africa. *Water* **1994**, *20*, 9–13.
30. Lindell, M.K.; Perry, R.W. Household Adjustment to Earthquake Hazard: A Review of Research. *Environ. Behav.* **2000**, *32*, 461–501. [CrossRef]
31. Biernacki, W.; Dziaek, J.; Janas, K.; Pado, T. *Community Attitudes towards Extreme Phenomena Relative to Place of Residence and Previous Experience*; Łódzkie Towarzystwo Naukowe: Łódź, Poland, 2008.
32. Wachinger, G.; Renn, O.; Begg, C.; Kuhlicke, C. The Risk Perception Paradox-Implications for Governance and Communication of Natural Hazards. *Risk Anal.* **2013**, *33*, 1049–1065. [CrossRef]
33. Xu, D.; Qing, C.; Deng, X.; Yong, Z.; Ma, Z. Disaster Risk Perception, Sense of Pace, Evacuation Willingness, and Relocation Willingness of Rural Households in Earthquake-Stricken Areas: Evidence from Sichuan Province, China. *Int. J. Environ. Res. Public Health* **2020**, *17*, 602. [CrossRef]
34. Xue, K.; Xu, D.; Liu, S. Social Network Influences on Non-Agricultural Employment Quality for Part-Time Peasants: A Case Study of Sichuan Province, China. *Sustainability* **2019**, *11*, 4134. [CrossRef]
35. Fiore, J.; Becker, J.; Coppel, D.B. Social network interactions: A buffer or a stress. *Am. J. Community Psychol.* **1983**, *11*, 423–439. [CrossRef] [PubMed]
36. Inkpen, A.C.; Tsang, E.W.K. Social capital, networks, and knowledge transfer. *Acad. Manag. Rev.* **2005**, *30*, 146–165. [CrossRef]
37. Jones, E.C.; Faas, A.J.; Murphy, A.; Tobin, G.A.; Mccarty, C. *Social Networks and Disaster Risk Perception in Mexico and Ecuador*; Springer International Publishing: Cham, Switzerland, 2018; pp. 151–166.
38. Koku, E.; Felsher, M. The Effect of Social Networks and Social Constructions on HIV Risk Perceptions. *Aids Behav.* **2020**, *24*, 206–221. [CrossRef]
39. Reininger, B.M.; Rahbar, M.H.; Lee, M.; Chen, Z.X.; Alam, S.R.; Pope, J.; Adams, B. Social capital and disaster preparedness among low income Mexican Americans in a disaster prone area. *Soc. Sci. Med.* **2013**, *83*, 50–60. [CrossRef] [PubMed]
40. Han, Z.; Wang, L.; Cui, K. Trust in stakeholders and social support: Risk perception and preparedness by the Wenchuan earthquake survivors. *Environ. Hazards* **2020**, *10*, 1–14. [CrossRef]
41. Terpstra, T. *Flood Preparedness: Thoughts, Feelings and Intentions of the Dutch Public*; University of Twente: Enskod, The Netherlands, 2009.
42. Lianjiang, L. Political Trust in Rural China. *Mod. China* **2016**, *30*, 228–258. [CrossRef]
43. Ponzo, M.; Scoppa, V. The use of informal networks in Italy: Efficiency or favoritism? *J. Behav. Exp. Econ.* **2010**, *39*, 89–99. [CrossRef]
44. Liu, S.Q.; Xie, F.T.; Zhang, H.Q.; Guo, S.L. Influences on rural migrant workers' selection of employment location in the mountainous and upland areas of Sichuan, China. *J. Rural Stud.* **2014**, *33*, 71–81. [CrossRef]
45. Xu, D.; Guo, S.; Xie, F.; Liu, S.; Cao, S. The impact of rural laborer migration and household structure on household land use arrangements in mountainous areas of Sichuan Province, China. *Habitat Int.* **2017**, *70*, 72–80. [CrossRef]
46. Xie, F.; Liu, S.-Q.; Xu, D. Gender difference in time-use of off-farm employment in rural Sichuan, China. *J. Rural Stud.* **2019**. [CrossRef]

47. Xu, D.; Zhuang, L.M.; Deng, X.; Qing, C.; Yong, Z.L. Media Exposure, Disaster Experience, and Risk Perception of Rural Households in Earthquake-Stricken Areas: Evidence from Rural China. *Int. J. Env. Res. Public Health* **2020**, *17*, 3246. [CrossRef] [PubMed]
48. Xu, D.; Deng, X.; Kai, H.; Liu, Y.; Yong, Z.; Liu, S.-Q. Relationships between labor migration and cropland abandonment in rural China from the perspective of village types. *Land Use Policy* **2019**, *88*, 104164. [CrossRef]
49. Xu, D.; Yong, Z.L.; Deng, X.; Liu, Y.; Huang, K.; Zhou, W.F.; Ma, Z.X. Financial Preparation, Disaster Experience, and Disaster Risk Perception of Rural Households in Earthquake-Stricken Areas: Evidence From the Wenchuan and Lushan Earthquakes in China's Sichuan Province. *Int. J. Env. Res. Public Health* **2019**, *16*, 3345. [CrossRef] [PubMed]
50. Xu, D.; Liu, E.; Wang, X.; Hong, T.; Liu, S. Rural Households' Livelihood Capital, Risk Perception, and Willingness to Purchase Earthquake Disaster Insurance: Evidence from Southwestern China. *Int. J. Environ. Res. Public Health* **2018**, *15*, 1319. [CrossRef] [PubMed]
51. Johnston, D.; Paton, D.; Crawford, G.L.; Ronan, K.; Houghton, B.; Burgelt, P. Measuring tsunami preparedness in coastal Washington, United States. *Nat. Hazards* **2005**, *35*, 173–184. [CrossRef]
52. Yang, J.; Yang, Y.B.; Liu, X.F.; Tian, J.Q.; Zhu, X.; Miao, D.M. Self-efficacy, social support, and coping strategies of adolescent earthquake survivors in china. *Soc. Behav. Pers.* **2010**, *38*, 1219–1228. [CrossRef]
53. Murray, M.; Watson, P.K. Adoption of natural disaster preparedness and risk reduction measures by business organisations in Small Island Developing States-A Caribbean case study. *Int. J. Disaster Risk Reduct.* **2019**, *39*, 12. [CrossRef]
54. Adeola, F.O. Katrina Cataclysm Does Duration of Residency and Prior Experience Affect Impacts, Evacuation, and Adaptation Behavior Among Survivors? *Env. Behav.* **2009**, *41*, 459–489. [CrossRef]
55. Durage, S.W.; Kattan, L.; Wirasinghe, S.C.; Ruwanpura, J.Y. Evacuation behaviour of households and drivers during a tornado. *Nat. Hazards* **2014**, *71*, 1495–1517. [CrossRef]
56. Lim, M.B.B.; Lim, H.R.; Piantanakulchai, M.; Uy, F.A. A household-level flood evacuation decision model in Quezon City, Philippines. *Nat. Hazards* **2016**, *80*, 1539–1561. [CrossRef]
57. Lazega, E.; Wasserman, S.; Faust, K. Social network analysis: Methods and applications. *Rev. Franaise Sociol.* **1995**, *36*, 781–783. [CrossRef]
58. Acock, A.C. Social networks, marital status, and well-being. *Soc. Netw.* **1993**, *15*, 309–334. [CrossRef]
59. Borgatti, S. Social Network Analysis, Two-Mode Concepts in. *Comput. Complex. Theory Tech. Appl.* **2009**. [CrossRef]
60. Heaney, C.A.; Israel, B.A. *Social Networks and Social Support*; Springer: New York, NY, USA, 2009; pp. 189–210, ISBN 978-0-387-75888-6.
61. Jack, S.L. The Role, Use and Activation of Strong and Weak Network Ties: A Qualitative Analysis. *J. Manag. Stud.* **2010**, *42*, 1233–1259. [CrossRef]
62. Louch, H. Personal network integration: Transitivity and homophily in strong-tie relations. *Soc. Netw.* **2000**, *22*, 45–64. [CrossRef]
63. Wendy, M. Providing Affective Information to Family and Friends Based on Social Networks. In Proceedings of the CHI 2007 Conference on Human Factors in Computing Systems, San Jose, CA, USA, 28 April–3 May 2007; pp. 2219–2224.
64. Borgatti, S.; Jones, C.; Everett, M. Network measures of social capital. *Connections* **1998**, *21*, 1–36.
65. Lin, N. A Network Theory of Social Capital. *Connect* **1998**, *22*, 8279–8291.
66. Borgatti, S.; Li, X. On Social Network Analysis in a Supply Chain Context. *J. Supply Chain Manag.* **2009**, *45*, 5–22. [CrossRef]
67. Scherer, C.W.; Cho, H. A Social Network Contagion Theory of Risk Perception. *Risk Anal.* **2003**, *23*, 261–267. [CrossRef]
68. Hu, R. Chinese Rural Residents' Wedding and Funeral Networks and Their Influencing Factors. *Sociol. Rev. China* **2013**, *1*, 49–58. (In Chinese)
69. Zhang, L. *Study on Social Networks' Impact on the Wages of Migrant Workers*; Jinan University: Guangzhou, China, 2016. (In Chinese)
70. McAllister, D.J. Affect-based and cognition-based trust as foundations for interpersonal cooperation in organizations. *Acad. Manag. J.* **1995**, *38*, 24–59. [CrossRef]
71. Luo, J.W.; Luo, H.M.; Yan, C.K. *The Research on Consumers' Cognition Trust and Affeciton Trust in Network Retailers*; Publishing House Electronics Industry: Beijing, China, 2008; pp. 170–173.
72. Lee, J.; Lee, J.N.; Tan, B.C.Y. Emotional Trust and Cognitive Distrust: From A Cognitive-Affective Personality System Theory Perspective. In Proceedings of the Pacific Asia Conference on Information Systems, PACIS 2010, Taipei, Taiwan, 9–12 July 2010.
73. Ahsan, D.A. Does natural disaster influence people's risk preference and trust? An experiment from cyclone prone coast of Bangladesh. *Int. J. Disaster Risk Reduct.* **2014**, *9*, 48–57. [CrossRef]
74. Han, Z.; Xiaoli, L.; Elisa, I.; Hörhager, J.Y. The effects of trust in government on earthquake survivors' risk perception and preparedness in China. *Nat. Hazards* **2017**, *86*, 437–452. [CrossRef]
75. Schaubroeck, J.; Lam, S.S.K.; Peng, A.C.Y. Cognition-Based and Affect-Based Trust as Mediators of Leader Behavior Influences on Team Performance. *J. Appl. Psychol.* **2011**, *96*, 863–871. [CrossRef] [PubMed]
76. Mayo, R. Cognition is a matter of trust: Distrust tunes cognitive processes. *Eur. Rev. Soc. Psychol.* **2015**, *26*, 283–327. [CrossRef]
77. Armas, I. Earthquake Risk Perception in Bucharest, Romania. *Risk Anal.* **2006**, *26*, 1223–1234. [CrossRef]
78. Kellens, W.; Zaalberg, R.; Neutens, T.; Vanneuville, W.; De Maeyer, P. An Analysis of the Public Perception of Flood Risk on the Belgian Coast. *Risk Anal.* **2011**, *31*, 1055–1068. [CrossRef] [PubMed]
79. Miller, E.; Buys, L. The impact of social capital on residential water-affecting behaviors in a drought-prone Australian community. *Soc. Nat. Resour.* **2008**, *21*, 244–257. [CrossRef]

80. Babcicky, P.; Seebauer, S. The two faces of social capital in private flood mitigation: Opposing effects on risk perception, self-efficacy and coping capacity. *J. Risk Res.* **2016**, *20*, 1017–1037. [CrossRef]
81. Wu, X.H.; Li, X.G. Effects of Mass Media Exposure and Social Network Site Involvement on Risk Perception of and Precautionary Behavior Toward the Haze Issue in China. *Int. J. Commun.* **2017**, *11*, 3975–3997.
82. Vigoda-Gadot, E.; Talmud, I. Organizational Politics and Job Outcomes: The Moderating Effect of Trust and Social Support. *J. Appl. Soc. Psychol.* **2010**, *40*, 2829–2861. [CrossRef]
83. Nunkoo, R.; Ramkissoon, H. Power, trust, social exchange and community support. *Ann. Tour. Res.* **2012**, *39*, 997–1023. [CrossRef]
84. Dunning, D.; Fetchenhauer, D.; Schlosser, T.M. Trust as a social and emotional act: Noneconomic considerations in trust behavior. *J. Econ. Psychol.* **2012**, *33*, 686–694. [CrossRef]
85. Wu, J.-J.; Khan, H.A.; Chien, S.-H.; Lee, Y.-P. Impact of Emotional Support, Informational Support, and Norms of Reciprocity on Trust Toward the Medical Aesthetic Community: The Moderating Effect of Core Self-Evaluations. *Interact. J. Med. Res.* **2019**, *8*, e11750. [CrossRef] [PubMed]
86. Zhang, M.H.; Zhong, J.N.; Su, Y. Trust in Local Ability of Reducing Disasters and its Influences on Public Flood Risk Perception: Based on the Investigation and Analysis. In *Theory and Practice of Risk Analysis and Crisis Response, Proceedings*; Huang, C., Liu, X., Eds.; Atlantis Press: Paris, France, 2008; pp. 345–350.
87. Armaş, I.; Avram, E. Perception of flood risk in Danube Delta, Romania. *Nat. Hazards* **2009**, *50*, 269–287. [CrossRef]
88. Grayscholz, D.; Haney, T.J.; Macquarrie, P. Out of Sight, Out of Mind? Geographic and Social Predictors of Flood Risk Awareness. *Risk Anal.* **2019**, *39*, 2543–2558. [CrossRef] [PubMed]
89. Chen, R.; Cui, P. Current Situation and Prospect of Community-based Disaster Risk Management. *J. Catastrophology* **2013**, *28*, 133–138. [CrossRef]
90. Xi, Z.; Yi, L.; Dong, Z. Community-based disaster management: A review of progress in China. *Nat. Hazards* **2013**, *65*, 2215–2239. [CrossRef]
91. Ter Huurne, E.F.J.; Gutteling, J.M. How to trust? The importance of self-efficacy and social trust in public responses to industrial risks. *J. Risk Res.* **2009**, *12*, 809–824. [CrossRef]
92. Bernardo, F. Impact of place attachment on risk perception: Exploring the multidimensionality of risk and its magnitude. El impacto del apego al lugar sobre la percepción de riesgo: Explorando la multidimensionalidad del riesgo y su magnitud. *Estud. Psicol.* **2013**, *34*, 323–329. [CrossRef]
93. Bronfman, N.C.; Cisternas, P.C.; Lopez-Vazquez, E.; Cifuentes, L.A. Trust and risk perception of natural hazards: Implications for risk preparedness in Chile. *Nat. Hazards* **2016**, *81*, 307–327. [CrossRef]
94. Lindell, M.K.; Hwang, S.N. Households' perceived personal risk and responses in a multihazard environment. *Risk Anal.* **2008**, *28*, 539–556. [CrossRef] [PubMed]
95. Xu, D.; Peng, L.; Su, C.; Liu, S.; Wang, X.; Chen, T. Influences of mass monitoring and mass prevention systems on peasant households' disaster risk perception in the landslide-threatened Three Gorges Reservoir area, China. *Habitat Int.* **2016**, *58*, 23–33. [CrossRef]
96. Ardaya, A.B.; Evers, M.; Ribbe, L. What influences disaster risk perception? Intervention measures, flood and landslide risk perception of the population living in flood risk areas in Rio de Janeiro state, Brazil. *Int. J. Disaster Risk Reduct.* **2017**, *25*, 227–237. [CrossRef]
97. Tanner, A.; Arvai, J. Perceptions of Risk and Vulnerability Following Exposure to a Major Natural Disaster: The Calgary Flood of 2013. *Risk Anal.* **2018**, *38*, 548–561. [CrossRef] [PubMed]

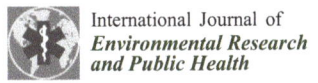

Article

The Impact of Individual Behaviors and Governmental Guidance Measures on Pandemic-Triggered Public Sentiment Based on System Dynamics and Cross-Validation

Hainan Huang [1], Weifan Chen [2], Tian Xie [1,*], Yaoyao Wei [1], Ziqing Feng [1] and Weijiong Wu [3]

[1] School of Economics, Management and Law at the University of South China, Hengyang 421001, China; hhn0113@outlook.com (H.H.); 2014002159@usc.edu.cn (Y.W.); fzq@stu.usc.edu.cn (Z.F.)

[2] Information Sciences and Technology at The Pennsylvania State University, State College, PA 16802, USA; weifan@psu.edu

[3] School of Management, Guangdong University of Technology, Guangzhou 510520, China; wuweijiong@gdut.edu.cn

* Correspondence: thanksky709394@163.com

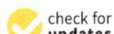

Citation: Huang, H.; Chen, W.; Xie, T.; Wei, Y.; Feng, Z.; Wu, W. The Impact of Individual Behaviors and Governmental Guidance Measures on Pandemic-Triggered Public Sentiment Based on System Dynamics and Cross-Validation. *Int. J. Environ. Res. Public Health* **2021**, *18*, 4245. https://doi.org/10.3390/ijerph18084245

Academic Editor: Paul B. Tchounwou

Received: 11 March 2021
Accepted: 14 April 2021
Published: 16 April 2021

Publisher's Note: MDPI stays neutral with regard to jurisdictional claims in published maps and institutional affiliations.

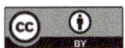

Copyright: © 2021 by the authors. Licensee MDPI, Basel, Switzerland. This article is an open access article distributed under the terms and conditions of the Creative Commons Attribution (CC BY) license (https://creativecommons.org/licenses/by/4.0/).

Abstract: Negative online public sentiment generated by government mishandling of pandemics and other disasters can easily trigger widespread panic and distrust, causing great harm. It is important to understand the law of public sentiment dissemination and use it in a timely and appropriate way. Using the big data of online public sentiment during the COVID-19 period, this paper analyzes and establishes a cross-validation based public sentiment system dynamics model which can simulate the evolution processes of public sentiment under the effects of individual behaviors and governmental guidance measures. A concrete case of a violation of relevant regulations during COVID-19 epidemic that sparked public sentiment in China is introduced as a study sample to test the effectiveness of the proposed method. By running the model, the results show that an increase in government responsiveness contributes to the spread of positive social sentiment but also promotes negative sentiment. Positive individual behavior suppresses negative emotions while promoting the spread of positive emotions. Changes in the disaster context (epidemic) have an impact on the spread of sentiment, but the effect is mediocre.

Keywords: pandemic; public sentiment; system dynamics; cross-validation; simulation and control

1. Introduction

In January 2020, an outbreak of COVID-19 began in Wuhan, China; this virus eventually spread rapidly to more than 200 countries. Since then, there have been over 79.2 million cases and 1.7 million deaths reported [1]. Closing educational institutions and face-to-face businesses, limiting gatherings to 10 people or less, and strict stay-at-home orders are many non-pharmaceutical interventions (NPIs) that governments put in place in an attempt to control the COVID-19 pandemic. However, NPIs can also indirectly create new problems: negative public sentiment and misinformation.

During the period of home quarantine, physical interpersonal communication is blocked and social networks become an essential communication channel. Due to the single source of information and fear of unknown viruses, a large number of negative online public sentiment incidents and misinformation spreading broke out during the pandemic, such as the Shuang-huang-lian panic buying incident in China, the 5G-caused spread of coronavirus in the UK, and more. Past empirical research results have shown that public health emergencies can trigger more negative public sentiment and misinformation, generating negative emotions and affecting psychological and physical health. Negative emotions may damage the immune system, leading to long-term infections and delayed wound healing [2]. During an epidemic, if the government fails to guide public xenophobia, it may lead to public blame of the government [3] (e.g., black Africans blaming

AIDS(Acquired Immune Deficiency Syndrome) on the white governments of non-African countries [4,5]), and people who do not trust the government may not participate in beneficial public health programs (e.g., government-mandated vaccination programs [6–8]). Based on the above research conclusions, how to guide the negative public sentiment in time and improve the individual's emergency psychology preparedness is the central topic of the research.

The study of negative public sentiment and misinformation usually uses an empirical and model-based approach. Public emotions and cognition are usually measured by retrospective questionnaires, such as the Oxford Happiness Inventory [9], Symptom Checklist 90 [10] and Likert Type Attitude Scale [11]. Using scales, questionnaires, and second-hand data to build statistical models is an important method for analyzing public psychology. On the one hand, a large number of scholars have studied the influence of public sentiment on the external factors. For example, Gilles et al. found that public trust in medical organizations was related to vaccination behavior and predicted the public's H1N1(2009 swine flu pandemic) vaccination behavior in 2009 [7]. Bogart et al. found a strong relationship between AIDS conspiracy and medical non-adherence among African Americans [6]. Hong et al. revealed the relationship between public trust in the government and individual public health emergency preparedness [12]. On the other hand, many scholars have studied the intrinsic generation and evolutionary logic of public emotions. For example, Li et al. used social platform data to study the evolution of public psychology before and after the declaration of the COVID-19 epidemic [13]. Apuke et al. analyzed the internal motivation of sharing fake news from psychological factors such as "altruism", "entertainment", and "socialization", based on the Uses and Gratification framework [14]. Hong et al. studied the relationship between political news in different forms of media and public happiness psychology [15]. Differing from empirical research, model-based research focuses on public psychology prediction, policy evaluation, communication mechanism, complex system behavior, etc., and have unique advantages in considering complex, nonlinear, and self-loop. For example, Liu et al. established a contagion diffusion model for public opinion simulation based on game theory to reveal the contagion path of public opinion [16]. Naskar et al. studied the public sentiment propagation characteristics of Twitter users based on the Russell model and TESC technology [17]. Xie et al. proposed a parallel evolution and response decision-making framework of public emotion based on system dynamics and parallel control management theories, which is a real-time decision-making method to simulate and control public sentiment [18].

A review of literature in recent years reveals that many fields, including public health [13], business management [19], medical management [7], communication media [17], emergency management [18], and economics [20] have conducted research on public psychology, but there is still a certain lack in model construction, validation, and applicable measures analysis. Considering that a single linear model is not sufficient to reflect the real social complex system of nonlinear multiple information and self-feedback, a system dynamics method is introduced on the basis of the linear model, so as to consider the nonlinear characteristics and avoid the subjectivity of the parameter. In addition, considering the lack of data and the model validation, we introduce the cross-validation method to improve the effectiveness of the model. Finally, considering the stochastic characteristics of the real world, this article introduces a random process on the basis of the model to make the model more suitable for real situations. Figure 1 shows the research idea map of this article.

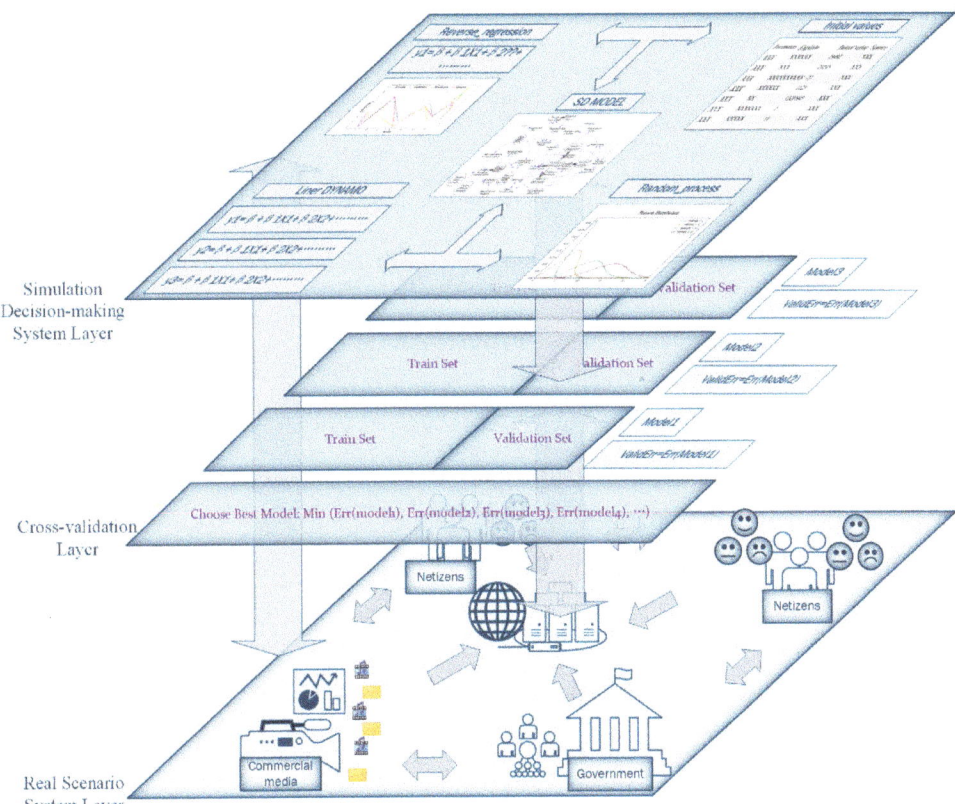

Figure 1. Cross-validation modeling framework for public sentiment system.

2. Materials and Methods

2.1. Cross-Validation Modeling Framework for Public Sentiment Based on System Dynamics

Cross-validation is a model selection method that can be used to directly estimate Generalization Error. This method can be used for model verification and model effectiveness improving. Because of its simplicity, it is widely used in the machine learning field [21,22]. Usually, the internal relationships of a public sentiment system, which describe the operating rules and determine the validity of simulation results, are difficult to verify. Therefore, the "Cross-validation modeling framework for public sentiment based on system dynamics" (CVMFPS) is proposed as a guideline to solve this problem (Figure 1). According to the "scenario-response"-based emergency management paradigm [23], and combined with the cross-validation method, this model consists of three parts: the real scenario system layer, the cross-validation layer, and the simulation decision-making layer.

2.1.1. Real Scenario System Layer

As the source of information, real scenarios are the basis for decision-making as well as the targets of public sentiment control. The original events, sentiment disseminators and sentiment regulators are essential elements of the real scenario system. The original events (such as public health emergencies, government scandals and mistakes) may easily trigger relevant public sentiment. Public sentiment disseminators include the media, netizens, and others. The media triggers and influences the processes of public sentiment propagation through reporting and directing the news. In addition, netizens use social networks to express and communicate their own opinions which results in the continued diffusion and evolution of public sentiments. Because collective behaviors of the netizens comprehensively effect their attitudes towards source events, their support or opposition are essential factors for the government in making an efficient response decision. Generally, the government response departments dealing with the emergencies or mistakes assume the greatest responsibilities as public sentiment regulators. By taking measures such as holding lectures and seminars, press conferences on the events, and by releasing positive news, they may supervise, guide, and even control the development of the public sentiments.

2.1.2. Cross-Validation Layer

Using data for training model without testing, even if training error is small, does not mean that the model is correct. The model fits well on the training set, but the actual predictions are poor due to overfitting problems. In order to overcome this problem, the cross-validation method was proposed. The idea of this method is to divide the complete data set D (Equation (1)) into two parts randomly according to a certain proportion. The data set used to train the model is called the training set D^t (Equation (3)), and the data set used to test the model is called the validation set D^v (Equation (2)). In the Equations, s(1) represents the first data that output randomly, m represents the data size of the validation set, and n represents the total number of data sets. Since the training data and the validation data are not the same, the generalization error of the model is estimated on new data, and it is closer to the real generalization error. In the System Dynamics model, the dynamo equation reflecting the specific influence relationship between variables is constructed in a mathematical way, but due to the complexity, randomness and instability of the social system, the dynamo equation cannot be like accurately calculated like a physical model, so the quantitative relationship and directional relationship between the variables reflected by the dynamo equation under the social system need to be verified. Therefore, through the combination of variables, different internal model structures and mathematical equations are constructed, the cross-validation method is used to calculate the error of these models on the verification set and select the best model that is closest to the real situation, and this is an effective way to build models when the data is insufficient:

$$D = \{D_1, D_2, D_3, D_4 \ldots D_n\}, D = D^t + D^v \tag{1}$$

$$D^v = \{D_{s(1)}, D_{s(2)}, D_{s(3)}, D_{s(4)} \ldots D_{s(m)}\} \tag{2}$$

$$D^t = \{D_{s(m+1)}, D_{s(m+2)}, D_{s(m+3)}, D_{s(m+4)} \ldots D_{s(n)}\} \tag{3}$$

2.1.3. Simulation Decision-Making System Layer

From the cross-validation layer, we have well-structured system dynamics internal structures and dynamo equations. The dynamo equation is used to represent the specific relationship between various variables in the SD model. By adding stochastic process to dynamo equations, the SD model can evolve autonomously based on the random results at each time, its simulation results will be closer to reality, and the use of stochastic process can also test the robustness of the SD model. For example, the Poisson distribution can represent the frequency of occurrences of random events in a unit time and plug in each occurrence node, the mean frequency of occurrences of events in a unit time can be the parameter for Poisson distribution. In addition, this layer proposes a method to improve the simulation effect of the model, called Reverse Regression, which is different from linear regression (Equation (4)), the variable (*sharefactor*) in reverse regression (Equation (5)) does not have real data, this variable needs to be calculated by other independent variables and dependent variable. Reverse regression requires the *sharedfactor* to be constant during a certain event but change in different events, and also requires other variables (*othervar$_i$*) and *sharefactor* can explain the main variance of y. Therefore, by iterating the *sharedfactor* data, the trend of the *sharefactor* between different subjects tends to be consistent, and the value of the *sharedfactor* can be calculated. The specific calculation process is given in Section 3.2. Finally, by inputting the initial parameters of the new public sentiment event from the real scenario system and using these methods, the final SD model can be established. Through simulation, different response strategies or policies can be tested, verified, and optimized in the simulated environment

$$y = β_0 + β_1 * independent + β_i * othervar_i \quad (4)$$

$$y = β_0 + β_1 * sharedfactor + β_i * othervar_i \quad (5)$$

2.2. Methodology

Roadmaps are helpful for decision makers to know how to use a modelling and simulation method for dealing with practical problems [24]. To implement the CVMFPS method, we developed a roadmap that describes the steps shown in Figure 2. The order in the roadmap is only for reference, and we need to use the appropriate modeling order in the face of different real-world problems. In summary, the roadmap contains a series of steps, from data acquisition, modeling to simulation and analysis.

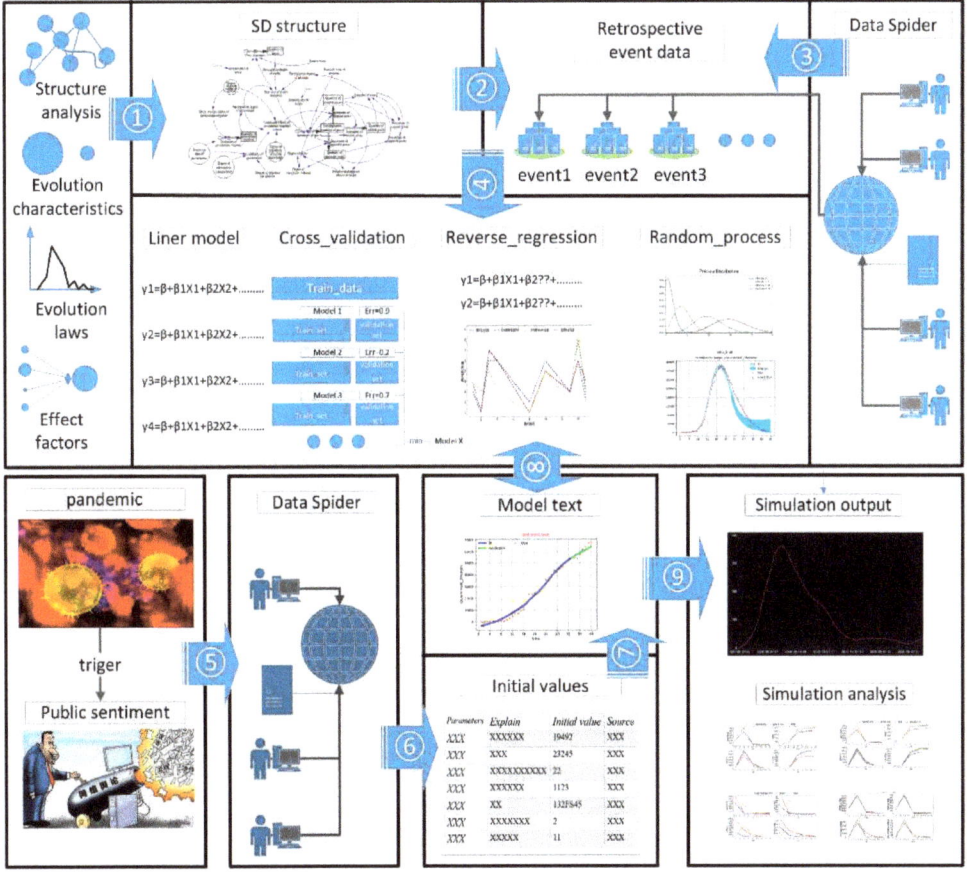

Figure 2. Research roadmap.

2.2.1. Decision Problem, Materials and Hypotheses

As a qualitative and quantitative decision-making method, the CVMFPS framework is applicable for response to the public sentiment without enough historical data. Therefore, the decision makers must determine what type of decision problem it is: Is there enough historical data for building a model for this event? If decision makers have enough investigable historical data, it is better to use the data-dependent statistical methods, such as Machine learning. If not, the SD (System Dynamics) simulation model with CVMFPS is a good idea. In addition, the source and measurement of data are also important issues to be considered before modeling, and for public sentiment, questionnaire data and secondary data are the main sources. There is a time lag for obtaining questionnaire data, which is often suitable for retrospective studies. Secondary data, especially the huge amount of data from social platforms, is easier to obtain and has great information potential, which is suitable for emergency research, but secondary data often has difficulty in data validation, and the common solution is to compare data from different data sources. In conclusion, it is particularly important to consider the type of data according to the model. For public sentiment, the use of web spider to obtain the latest data in real time on social networks is beneficial for SD model building and immediate policy analysis. Finally, the implementation of CVMFPS requires some prerequisite assumptions, and the fulfillment of which is a prerequisite for using the model. For public sentiment, CVMFPS often makes requirements in terms of the dissemination mechanism and simulation of sentiment.

2.2.2. SD Modelling

The SD emphasizes how causal relationships among system structures can influence the behaviors and evolution processes of a system. Analysis of the boundary and structure of a public sentiment system is the first step to building the SD model. System boundaries include the basic elements of the system. The function modules of the system consist of the elements that have direct causal relationships with each other.

System boundaries, influencing factors and causal loops are important for SD. Clarifying the system boundary of the problem facilitates us to focus on the subjects of the system without getting caught in the endless circulation of causal structures of complex social systems. In addition, the system boundary specifies the scope of application. The scope of application of the model is very important for practical applications; only when the important conditions are satisfied, the simulation results of the model have practical significance, and the focus of the model is consistent with the actual problem, is it possible to propose a solution strategy. The public sentiment system can be divided into original events and three interactional modules according to the different roles of the sentiment disseminators: the media module, the government module, and the netizen module. Therefore, the boundary of the public sentiment model should be within netizens, commercial media, and government. The purpose of the internal influence factor analysis of the system is to find out the relationship between each element. By distinguishing the independent and dependent variables, we can find a series of causal chains, and by transforming the dependent and independent variables, the influence is transmitted downward. When the lower end of the causal chain is connected to the upper end, the causal loop is thus generated [25]. The causal loop is the key to the autonomous evolution of the SD model, and the system has the ability to generate data autonomously when the effects of variables are fed back through different variables [26]. Usually, due to the wide distribution of Netizens and the profit-seeking nature of commercial media seeking exposure, these two types of subjects are the first to capture the events. The commercial media follows up on the events, the netizens express their opinions and generate emotions about them, and then, the stakeholders of the events (usually the government), depending on the nature of the events and the attitude of the public, responds accordingly. Moreover, the public, the commercial media, and the government will behave according to the behavior of other subjects, so interaction between the three types of subjects will form multiple causal loops that will eventually dominate the development of public sentiment.

Causal loop diagrams aid in visualizing a system's structure and behavior and in analyzing the system qualitatively. By analyzing the variables in the causal loop, we can construct more specific influence relationships, which will then involve specific mathematical formulas. To perform a more detailed quantitative analysis, a causal loop diagram is transformed into a stock and flow diagram. A stock is the term for any entity that accumulates or depletes over time, using an ordinary differential equation. A flow is the rate of change in a stock. In addition, in the stock flow paradigm, there are Auxiliary variables, relational linkages, etc. The judicious use of these tools will reduce the complexity of modeling. Moreover, it is also necessary to estimate the initial parameters. Usually, the parameters and initial conditions of the equations can be estimated using statistical methods, expert opinion, market research data, or other relevant sources of information [27]. Finally, converting the system stock flow paradigm into level, rate and auxiliary equations is the key step to run the model. In addition to constructing specific model structures and equations, we also nest random functions on equations. On the social network platform, the number of posts or reposts of netizens and media per unit time obeys a poisson distribution with λ as the mean value of posts. Therefore, for each time period, the number of posts of netizens or media is nested in a Poisson distribution (Equation (6)):

$$Posts = poisson\ (\lambda = mean(posts)) \qquad (6)$$

To construct specific mathematical equations, it is necessary to choose an appropriate expression method for the variable relationships. In complex social systems, the relationships between social variables cannot be constructed as precise equations can be constructed for engineering systems. Faced with the randomness, complexity, and incomplete predictability of social systems, it is a common and extremely practical method to estimate the relationships between variables in statistical models. There are quite a few statistical models that can reflect the relationship between variables, such as lin ear regression (LR), logistics regression, SVM (Support Vector Machine), neurl network, LSTM (Long Short-Term Memory), etc. The LR model is widely used by social science fields, such as economics and management. It is simple to operate and can predict continuous values. Although it is a linear model, the introduction of system dynamics can alleviate the linearity problem, so the LR model is used in this paper. Another purpose of using LR is to enable the reverse regression method. *Sharefactor* indicates that different variables are collectively influenced by *sharefactor*, and that *sharefactor* does not change within the same event (a short period of time) but change within different events (a long period of time). In the public sentiment system, the nature of the event itself (degree of harm to society, realistic fashion trends, etc.) and the nature of the netizens (education, income, family, etc.) will jointly influence the number of postings by netizens. The pseudo-code for the implementation process is detailed in Appendix A (Algorithm A1). The NRI in pseudocode 1 denotes the minimum times that the values in *sharefactor* are randomly varied so that the *othervar* and *sharefactor* variables can explain the main variance of the dependent variable. NI indicates how many sets of *sharefactor* are obtained; the larger the NI, the more likely it is to find the correct *sharefactor*, but there will be a large number of similar *sharefactors*. Pseudocode 1 finally outputs the most similar *sharefactor* between different dependent variables, and by drawing graphs of the *sharefactor* and observing the mutual trend, we can determine whether the *sharefactor* can be used or not. To obtain the value of *sharefactor* using linear regression, the following conditions need to be satisfied:

(1) The *sharefactor* values derived from different variables need to be verified against each other, and only if the trends are consistent can they be adopted;
(2) *Othervar* variables need to contain the main factors that can influence the dependent variable except *sharefactor*, i.e., *othervar* and *sharefactor* variables can explain the main variance of the dependent variable;
(3) Select the time period with less interference from external factors for reverse regression method, which facilitates the correct finding of *sharefactor* values;
(4) Assuming the value range of the *sharefactor* in advance, it is generally 0 to 10, −1 to 1 or 0 to 100, depending on requirements

2.2.3. Cross-Validation

When studying social problems, there are complex interactions within SD models, which make it impossible to construct accurate mathematical equations. When analyzing the independent variables of a dependent variable, we can't determine whether certain variables are independent or not. Reviewing the previous research results will identify some variables, but usually those are incomplete. The SD models constructed with incomplete variables will amplify the bias through feedback loops, which leads to unreliable simulation results. Therefore, we use the cross-validation method to select these uncertain variables and to verify the generalization ability of the mathematical equations. The pseudo-code for the implementation process is detailed in Appendix A (Algorithm A2). To run Algorithm A2, it is necessary to give the deterministic and uncertain variables in advance. One or more uncertain variables are selected at a time for regression on the basis of the deterministic variables. Then, the training set is used for training and the validation set is used to verify the training results. By adding different combinations of uncertain variables each time, we can get many models and select the model with the smallest validation set error as the mathematical model of SD. The data in the training and validation sets are in events as units, and each event is in units of time, so that when the data is split, the complete event, rather than the unit time of the events, can be used as the validation object. This allows for a better validation effect of the generalization ability of the model. Finally, the use of the cross-validation method also needs to satisfy the premise that the error of the model trained from the training set is small.

2.2.4. Simulating and Decision Analysis

Some advanced SD software tools, such as Vensim (Ventana Systems Inc., Harvard, MA, USA), STELLA (Isee Systems, Lebanon, PA, USA) and Anylogic (The AnyLogic Company, Oakbrook Terrace, IL, USA), are able to help decision-makers construct, run and analyze the SD simulation models of public sentiment systems to create optimized response policies and solutions in a graphic and visual way [28]. However, these software packages can have limited functions; if you want to apply new algorithms or use unique equations, they will need to be implemented using your own programming. To propose suitable response solutions, the relevant decision analysis process should include two aspects [18]. First, response strategies setting. In constructing the SD model, control variables need to be considered in advance, and for public sentiment, we can set control variables from three perspectives: public, government, and commercial media. The public side can be started from the personal side, such as education, science popularization, the degree of trust in the government, etc. The government side is variables such as response time, information transparency, science popularization, etc. Commercial media would be variables such as speed of reporting, dissemination, etc. In addition, we also need response strategy testing. The effects of different strategies can then be applied by reviewing the simulation results. By adjusting control variables, we can achieve the expected results.

2.3. Empirical Research

Roadmaps are helpful for decision makers to know how to use a modelling and simulation method for dealing with practical problems [24]. To implement the CVMFPS method, we developed a roadmap that describes the steps shown in Figure 2. The order in the roadmap is only for reference, and we need to use the appropriate modeling order in the face of different real-world problems. In summary, the roadmap contains a series of steps, from data acquisition, modeling to simulation and analysis.

2.3.1. Data Source

We used the top public sentiment events on Sina Weibo about COVID-19 from 25 January to 20 April 2020 in mainland China as samples [29]. The Sina Weibo contained more than 1.16 million active Weibo users. Weibo is a popular platform to share and discuss individual information and life activities, as well as celebrity news in China [30].

In this paper, we use third-party python libraries such as selenium, bs4 and urllib to write crawler programs to collect relevant data from government media, commercial media, and netizens, including the number of posts, blog ID(Identity document), the number of followers, posting content, the number of likes, number of comments, posting time, etc. A total of 15 online public sentiment events were collected during the period and used as historical cross-sectional data for equation construction within the SD model, the data description is shown by Table 1. In addition, we use the new event "Picked up the son from Wuhan to Jingzhou during the city closure", a local government official's epidemic prevention failure that occurred on February 14, as the simulation object of the SD model to test the feasibility and validity of the model. The data collected in this paper were cross-checked by Tencent WeChat subscriptions platform (Tencent, Shenzhen, China) [31] and the third-party ZhiWeiData platform (ZhiWeiData, Beijing, China) [32], and the results of the three-party data were consistent.

Table 1. Description of data.

Data Name	Pre-Response n (%)	Post-Response n (%)
Total posts	1,242,287 (57)	935,790 (43)
Total original posts	136,197 (56)	105,969 (44)
Total reposts	1,106,090 (57)	829,821 (43)
Total followers	197 billion (31)	439 billion (69)
Government original posts	3368 (30)	7944 (70)
Government reposts	295,853 (44)	382,303 (56)
Government followers	93 billion (27)	253 billion (73)
Commercial media original posts	15,003 (35)	28,032 (65)
Commercial media reposts	810,237 (64)	447,518 (36)
Commercial media followers	104 billion (36)	186 billion (64)
Netizen original posts	117,826 (63)	69,993 (37)

2.3.2. SD Modelling

The COVID-19 pandemic that broke out in early 2020 shattered the public's sense of normalcy. In the early stages of the outbreak, people used the Internet to keep an eye on the dynamics of the outbreak in the face of the rapidly spreading virus. During this period, several public sentiment incidents erupted on the internet, most of them as a response to government negligence or individual citizens not following orders. For example, a traveler who returned from Thailand did not comply with the epidemic prevention guidelines, Wuhan government officials failed to effectively ensure normal life for residents during home quarantine, etc. Taking these events as cases, we can analyze the boundary, structure and evolution mechanism of the public sentiment system and build a relevant qualitative causal loop diagram model. This model is divided into three main modules and two scenarios: the commercial media module, the netizen module, the government module, pre-response scenario, and post-response scenario.

System boundary and prerequisite assumptions. The interactions among three subjects—netizens, commercial media and government constitute the boundary of the public sentiment system, and factors outside of these subjects are not studied in this paper. In addition, this model requires the following prerequisites to be met:

(1) Public sentiment events are the first to erupt on the Internet.
(2) Different public sentiment events are independent of each other.
(3) When a negative event is revealed and not properly handled, the public will develop negative sentiment.
(4) Positive public sentiment will arise after the government actively and properly handles negative events.

The causal loop diagram of the SD model consists of three modules and two scenarios. The three modules include netizen, commercial media, and government. Netizens, commercial media, and government together constitute the total discussions online, while the herding and hotspot effects that exist in the spread of public sentiment cause discussions online to in turn promote the level of discussion among the three, thus forming multiple causal loops, as shown in Figure 3a. Netizens (commercial media and government) discussions and discussions online form a positive feedback loop. In addition, the two scenarios include pre-response and post-response scenarios. The government's response to the incident is a turning point in the development of public sentiment. After the government's response, netizens and commercial media turn their attention to the discussion of the content of the government's response. The government guides public sentiment by making the right measures and spreading positive information, so that post-response public sentiment communication also forms the same mechanism as the pre-response, and the causal loops are also positive feedback loop. Finally, post-response communication of public sentiment has an impact on pre-response communication and form a negative feedback loop.

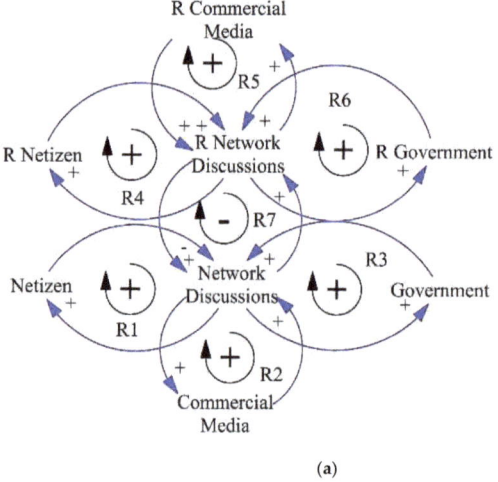

(a)

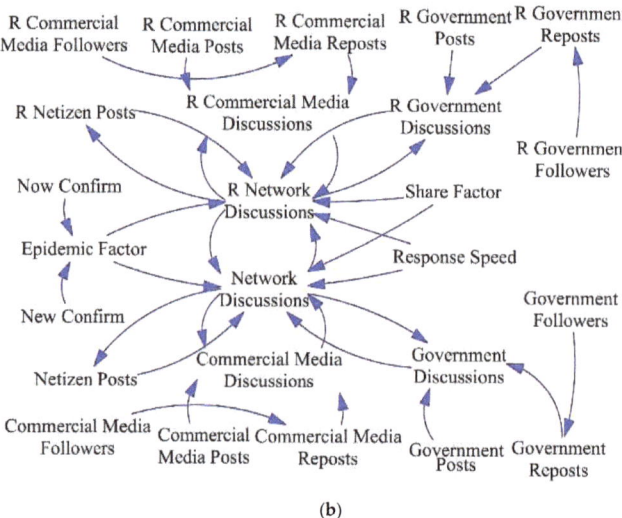

(b)

Figure 3. (a) Causal loop diagram of the public sentiment system; (b) Public sentiment transmission mechanism of social platforms.

Causal loop detailing and reverse regression. On the basis of the causal loop, we perform a causal analysis to each factor: looking for the constituents and independent variables. If necessary, further causal analysis of these independent variables and constituents can be performed. As a result, the previous causal loop is expanded into a more detailed loop diagram. In the process of detailing, it is necessary to determine the independent and dependent variables for each factor, and also to confirm whether the independent variables meet the *sharefactor* characteristics, the detailed causal loop diagram is shown in Figure 3b. Through the data, we found that most of the posts posted by netizens will not be reposted by others; in order to reduce complexity, we only consider their original posts. Commercial media includes original posts and reposts; the reposts are influenced by the number of followers of the blogger. Government media is the same as commercial media. In addition, we add Response Speed, Epidemic Factor and Share Factor in the loop. The Epidemic Factor takes into account the environmental disaster context, the Share Factor needs to be calculated by Reverse Regression, and the specific interpretation of the variables is given by Appendix A (Table A1). Compared to the middle and late period (There is a large number of non-linear relationships in middle and late periods) of an event development, in the early period public sentiment propagation mechanisms is much simpler. Therefore, we choose the first day of the event as the cross-section sample to run reverse regression, and choose netizen post, commercial media post, commercial media reports and government reposts as the cross-test subjects. Due to the fact that the first day data of some public sentiment events was missing, we selected nine events with intact data as samples. The reverse regression results are shown in Table 2 and Figure 4a. By observing Figure 4a, we can find highly similar trends among different subjects. Comparing the real data of these subjects (Figure 4b) shows that there is a high probability of finding the real *sharefactor*. Mean err in Table 2 is obtained by calculating the root mean square error of the two-by-two combination of the four subjects (Equation (7)). Where n denotes the number of samples and N denotes the number of the two-by-two combination of the four subjects. By averaging the *sharefactor* of these four subjects, the averaged *sharefactor* (Mean *sharefactor*) is used as the final result. The Mean *sharefactor* is then used to do a regression on a subject, and the resulting regression parameters can simplify the *sharefactor* calculation process for the new event (i.e., we only need the *othervar* and the dependent variables to calculate the *sharefactor* by these parameters):

$$CRMS = \frac{\sum_{j=1}^{N} \sqrt{\frac{\sum_{j=1}^{N}(y_{j1} - \hat{y}_{j2})^2}{n}}}{N} \tag{7}$$

Table 2. Reverse regression outcomes.

Name	Outcomes	*othervar*
Netizen Posts	[4,1,6,6,5,4,2,1,3,5,4.5,4,3,8,3]	RND, RS, EF
Commercial Media Posts	[3,1,7,6,5,4,3,2,4,6,5,4,3,6,2]	RND, RS, EF
Commercial Media Reposts	[4,3,5,3,2.5,2,1.5,1,3,5,4,3,2,9,2]	RND, RS, EF, CMF
Government Reposts	[4,1,7,6,5,4,2,1,3,5,4.5,4,3,6,4]	RND, RS, EF, GF
Mean err	1.85	-
Mean *sharefactor*	[3.75,1.5,6.25,5.25,4.375,3.5,2.125,1.25,3.25,5.25,4.5,3.75,2.75,7.25,2.75]	-
sharefactor equation [1]	NP = a + b * EF + c * SF + d * (RGP + RGR) a = −23328.98463791, b = 3273.79176234, c = 2080.23327003, d = 1002.55401367	-

[1] The equation uses "Netizen Posts" as the sample data and the abbreviations of the variables in the "Outcomes" column are given in Table A1.

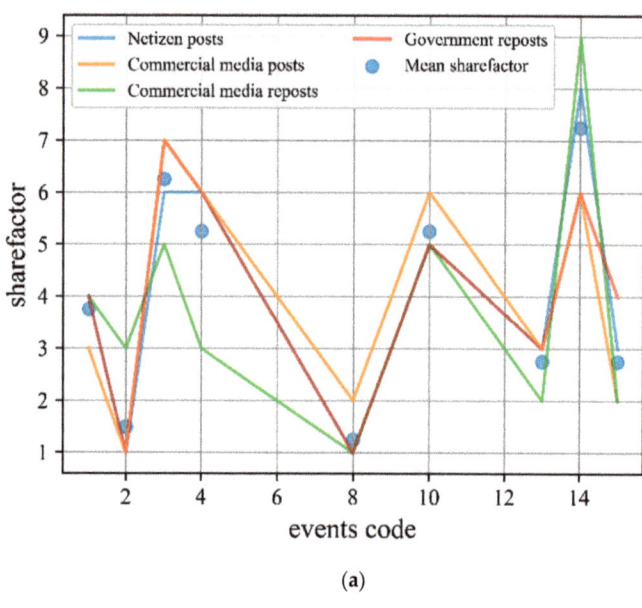

(a)

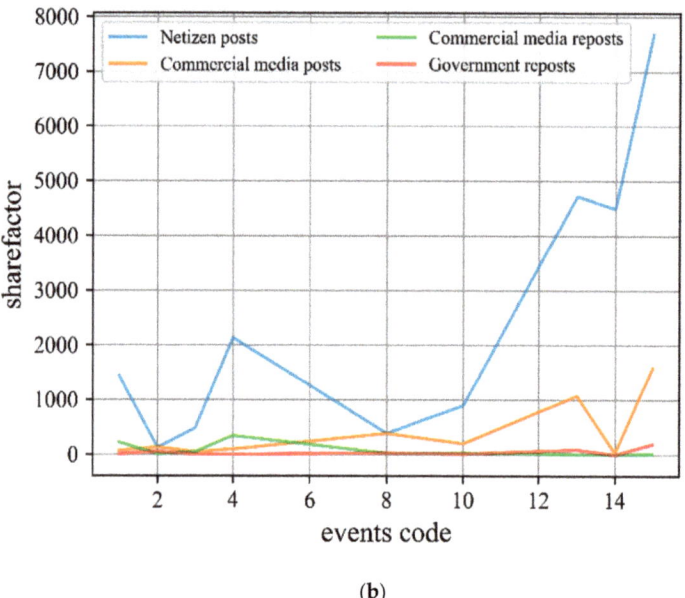

(b)

Figure 4. (**a**) Comparison of *sharefactor* trends between different subjects; (**b**) Comparison of raw data between different subjects.

2.3.3. Cross-Validation

After the variable analysis and data collection, the cross-validation method is applied to a total of 12 variables, and the specific process and results are shown in Table 3 and Figure 5. In general, variables that cannot be constructed by precise mathematical formulas (e.g., complex social factors) and cannot be controlled (e.g., the number of posts people make) need to be identified as dependent variables. The determination of independent variables requires an analysis of the impact relationship. At the same time, attention needs to be paid to the issue of the time sequence of occurrence, and variables that arise simultaneously or in the future cannot be included in independents. In addition, due to the error amplification effect of the causal feedback loop in the system, it is necessary to select the regression results with good training and validation GOF (Goodness of Fit) from the combination of independent variables, and the GOF of validation set can avoid the overfitting problem, the GOF of training set can reflect the validity of the model.

Table 3. Cross-validation process and results.

Dependent	Independent [1]	Train Set R2	Validation Set R2	Equations
NP	[RCMR, CMR, GF, RCMF, RNP, CMP, T, SF, RGR, GR, GFOC]	0.84	0.99	
CMP	[T, NP, SF, EF, GFOC]	0.99	0.97	
CMR	[T, BMP, RCMF, GP, GR, NP, CMF, SF, RGR, RNP, GF, RCMR, EF, GFOC]	0.86	0.97	
CMF	[T, BMP, GP, RCMF, GR, NP, SF, RCMP, RNP, GF, RCMR, EF, GFOC]	0.91	0.99	
GP	[BMP, T, NP, SF, EF, GFOC]	0.97	0.99	
GR	[BMP, T, RCMF, NP, SF, GF, EF, GFOC]	0.98	0.99	Table A1
GF	[BMP, T, RCMF, NP, SF, RCMP, RGR, CMR, RNP, RCMR, GFOC]	0.89	0.99	
RNP	[BMP, T, GP, GR, SF, RGR, RGP, CMR, EF]	0.97	0.99	
RCMP	[GP, SF, RGR, CMR, RGP, GF, EF, GFOC]	0.98	0.99	
RCMR	[T, BMP, RCMF, GP, GR, NP, SF, RGR, CMR]	0.86	0.98	
RCMF	[T, GP, GR, RGF, NP, SF, RGR, CMR, RGP, GF, EF, GFOC]	0.84	0.95	
RGR	[BMP, T, GR, NP, RGF, SF, CMR, GF, EF, GFOC]	0.95	0.99	

[1] the abbreviations of the variables in the "Independent" column are given in Table A1.

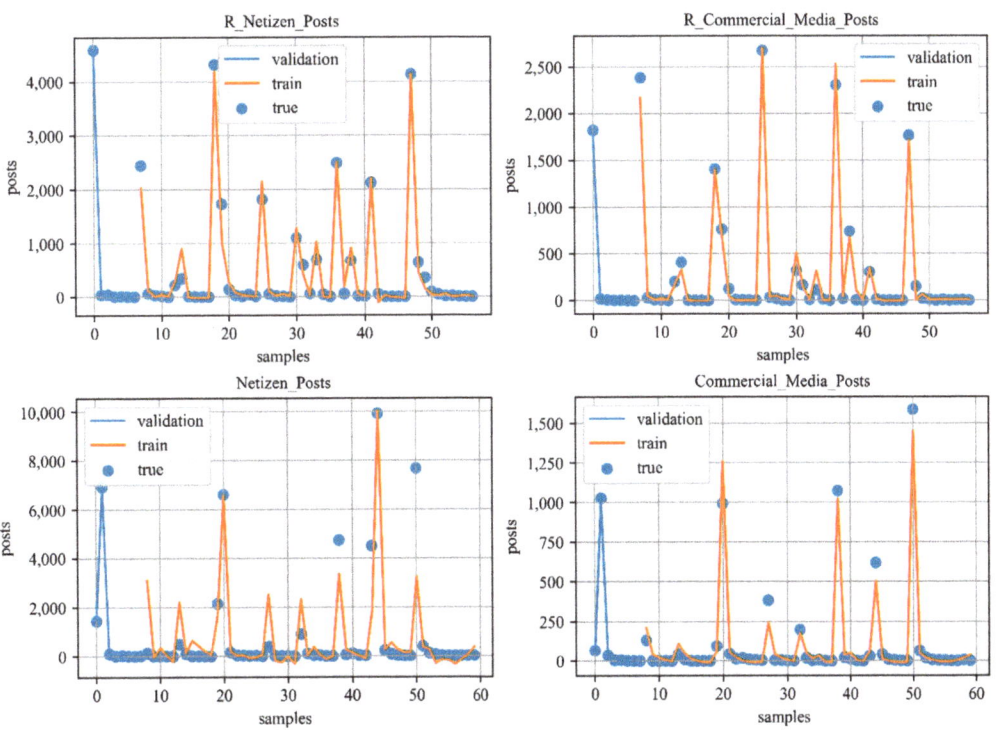

Figure 5. Partial training results and validation results.

positive individual behavior. However, the positive sentiment (R Network Discussions) curve is significantly higher than the baseline, with the cumulative number rising 207,036, proportional to the positive individual behavior. The amount of overall positive social public sentiment (Public Sentiment) increased by 219,561, and the overall social public sentiment is positive. Positive Netizen Strategy shows that positive individual behavior not only inhibits the spread of negative emotions, but also contributes more to the spread of positive emotions, which can increase the level of positive social public emotions in both directions. The simulation results of the "Negative Netizen Strategy" are the exact opposite of the "Positive Netizen Strategy": negative individual behavior not only increases the spread of negative emotions (18,292 more negative emotions), but also inhibits the spread of positive emotions (24,297 fewer positive emotions), which ultimately leads to a significant increase in overall negative social public sentiment. The opposite simulation results of "Positive Netizen Strategy" and "Negative Netizen Strategy" also verify the robustness of the model.

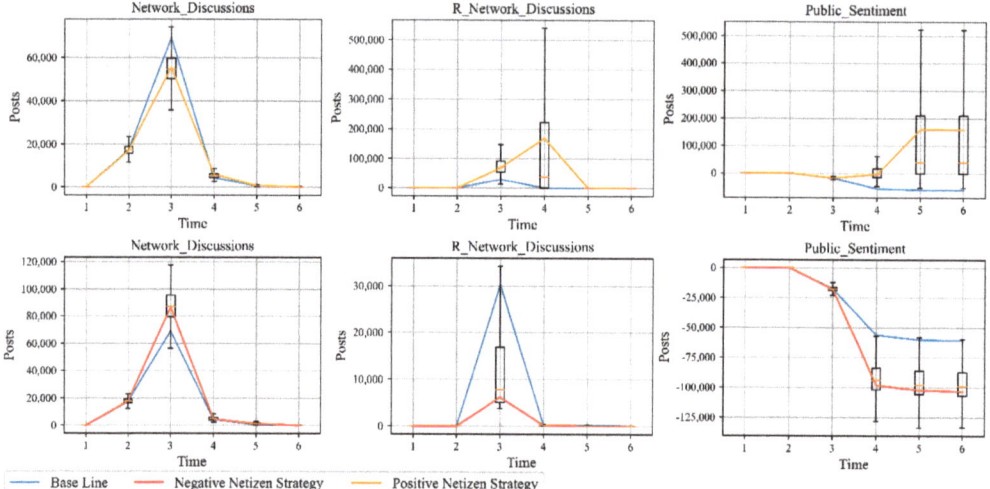

Figure 8. Netizen analysis.

As the main background of public opinion, disasters are the source of public sentiment events. To explore the impact of disaster context on the public sentiment system, we set the "Epidemic Strategy": Epidemic Factor increased by 40% to represent a worsening of the epidemic. The simulation results are shown in Figure 9 and Table 4. As the epidemic worsens, the negative sentiment curve is slightly higher than the baseline, proportional to the deterioration of the epidemic. The positive sentiment curve is slightly below the baseline, inversely proportional to the deterioration of the epidemic. Overall social sentiment has declined from the baseline. Although the simulation results all changed compared to the baseline, the magnitude of change was relatively small. This suggests that although disaster environments (epidemics) can have an effect on public sentiment, the effect is relatively mediocre.

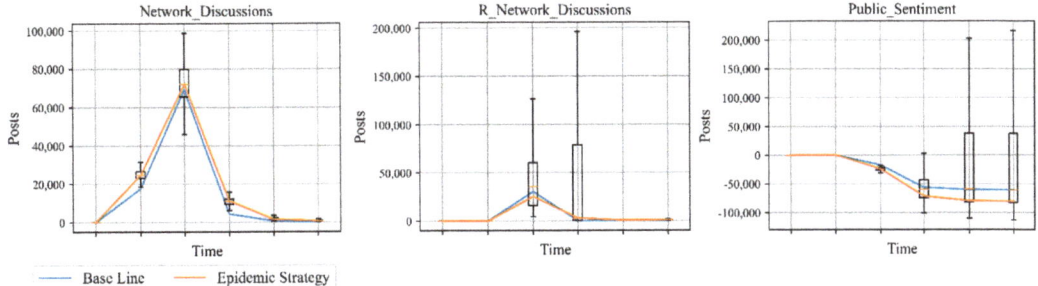

Figure 9. Epidemic analysis.

4. Discussion

According to the results of the model, we have reasons to believe that positive governmental response behavior is beneficial to redeem the positive image of the government among the public and even to reconstruct trust in the negative events derived from the epidemic. Specifically, the government uses e-government media to respond to negative events, and the strength of the government response represented by government postings and media influence can affect the spread of positive public sentiment. The strength of the government response is proportional to the number of positive emotions. Previous findings suggest that proactive actions by authorities can improve negative public sentiment and rumor management in emergency situations and yield positive social utility [33]. Enhancing public relations through social media has proven effective [34]. The simulation results in this paper again validate the above findings. According to Situational Crisis Communication Theory, under intentional crises or accidental crises (e.g., job failure, abuse of authority), rebuild strategies (e.g., aggressive crisis management, satisfactory compensation and punishment, creating an image of positive crisis management) are effective ways to recover or even rebuild reputation [35]. The results of this paper build on the rebuild strategies to further investigate the relationship between positive image promotion behaviors and the spread of positive emotions (reputation or trust). One possible explanation for why increased government responsiveness can facilitate the spread of positive sentiment is that the government, as a network leader, influences the public through high communication activity, credibility, network centrality, and the use of affective, assertive, and linguistic diversity in their online messages [36], and uses mass media to amplify public sentiment [37]. A study showed that exposure to HPV (Human Papilloma Virus) information was associated with the degree of HPV vaccination [38]. This suggests that the government communicates risk to the public through the repetition of information and emphasizes the good attitude of the government in dealing with negative events [39], thus the government has gained the trust of the people. Notably, we also found that government response strength was positively related to negative sentiment, which may seem odd, but similar results have been found in previous studies: higher average positive exposure intensity predicts decreased positive sentiment expression and increased negative sentiment expression [40]. A possible explanation is that the expansion of the scale of the same sentiment discussion might inhibit the expression of the same sentiment and favor a shift to the opposite sentiment [40]. In addition, the expanded scope of government response attracts the expression of negative sentiments from groups that are themselves distrustful of the government. Both explanations are plausible, but the exploration of specific causes and effects requires further research.

In both the Positive Netizen Strategy and the Negative Netizen Strategy, the conclusion is the same: positive individual behavior can inhibit the spread of negative emotions and promote the spread of positive emotions. Specifically, individuals who reduce the transmission of negative emotions and increase the transmission of positive emotions will contribute to an increase in positive social emotions. The results seem obvious, but the implications for the entire public sentiment system (including individuals, government, commercial media, context, etc.) are unknown and meaningful. Previous studies have shown that the formation of identical emotional groups is the result of two factors: emotional contagion and homophily (getting together with people of similar emotions) [41], with the former playing a major role [42]. The conclusion that emotions can be massively contagious on social networks has been extensively verified in previous studies [42–45], which is an almost confirmed fact, and our simulation results also prove this. Furthermore, previous empirical studies have shown that when individuals reduce their positive emotional expression of events, others' positive emotional expression decrease and negative expression increase accordingly [45]. This is consistent with the results of our individual behavioral simulations. This suggests that the emotional transmission results of individual behaviors may be related to the initial emotional distribution and the rate of emotional contagion. The final distribution of emotions depends on the distribution of initial emotions [46], and a higher number of individuals unaffected by the emotions of others can effectively reduce aggressive emotions and behaviors [47], and these results provide strong evidence for the influence of initial emotion distribution on emotional contagion. A deeper explanation for this is that strongly connected network structures (e.g., the influence or number of followers of an individual) satisfy the basic requirement for emotional contagion (the possibility of being more widely known) [43]. The contagion rate of emotions depends on the network structure, peer pressure, the nature of the emotion itself, and the characteristics of the individual. Research has shown that contagion of emotions is not only influenced by network structure, but also reinforces it (i.e., people are more willing to express views and empathy with people who have the same emotions) [43]. Peer pressure forces individuals with different emotions to switch to the same emotion. In addition, there are different findings on the contagiousness or influence of emotions in different research contexts. Some studies have suggested that negative emotions are more contagious compared to positive emotions [43,46], but others have taken the opposite view [48], while some have concluded that there is no significant difference in the contagiousness of different emotions [45]. In the Chinese situation, the government is more concerned with building its authority and credibility, so positive sentiment seems to be more popular with the public, as evidenced by the comparison of the effects of the Positive Netizen Strategy and the Negative Netizen Strategy. Finally, the effect of individual characteristics on emotional contagion is very rare in existing studies, but some side evidence suggests that individual personality type [49] (extrovert, introvert) and education [50] have a significant effect on emotional contagion.

Although the disaster context (epidemic) is the source of negative public sentiment events, our simulation results suggest that changes in the disaster context do not seem to have a significant enough impact on the spread of public sentiment. A worse disaster context after a negative event outbreak can slightly promote the spread of negative emotions and slightly inhibit the spread of positive emotions. To date, research on the context of emotional contagion has been relatively sparse, but many studies of sentiment analysis of social networks during COVID-19 seem to be able to detect some patterns. A Twitter analysis of Chinese Netizen sentiment during COVID-19 found that Chinese Netizens' sentiment was consistently negative, but increased slightly as the outbreak subsided [51]. In addition, many similar studies on Chinese microblogs (WeiBo, Sina, Beijing, China) have found similar results [52,53]. These studies were able to provide evidence for our results. One possible explanation for this result is that negative sentiment events are relatively independent of the disaster context once they are generated. The disaster context provides the initial conditions for the generation of negative emotional events, yet the spread of public sentiment relies heavily on emotional contagion. People are concerned about the problems exposed by the negative events and hope that the government can solve them properly. Therefore, the process of government handling and the process of people's emotional contagion are the main factors that affect public sentiment. Changes in the disaster context have the potential to influence public sentiment, but changes in the disaster context alone are not enough.

Currently, social media and e-government are playing an increasingly important role in exposing corruption and social problems [54]. It is a challenge for governments and institutions to rebuild their reputation while accepting beneficial improvements from the public. As mentioned at the beginning of this paper, people's trust in government or institutions plays a very important role in the acceptance of large beneficial public programs (e.g., vaccination). Therefore, we offer some suggestions and reflections based on the results of the study. Social media is a platform for presentation of the image of government, institutions, and local communities [55]. If official communication is marginalized or ignored, it will have serious consequences. As the speed of information interaction increases, governments and institutions first need to move from their former role as broadcasters to information participants and receivers [56]. Secondly, when the government informs the process of handling negative events, it needs to make announcements not only for the public, but also in terms of breadth and depth. Especially in the face of some negative events that may seriously damage the credibility, it is necessary not only to expand the range of users of the announcement as much as possible, but also to give more in-depth interpretations for different government or institutional media (e.g., legal, life, etc.). Finally, governments or institutions need to cultivate media with significant influence and authority over time. The role of these media in guiding sentiment, dispelling rumors, and rebuilding reputations is enormous.

The population is more inclined to follow the emotional expressions of the overall channel than the specific information content in social networks [41], which indicates that people's emotions can be easily manipulated maliciously. Reducing malicious manipulation of emotions requires both individual and institutional efforts. First of all, the content review mechanism of social media platforms needs to be improved, and comments that are obviously violent, discriminatory and anti-human need to be banned or alerted. Those negative messages that have not been confirmed also need to be informed to each recipient. The purpose of this is to reduce the degree of connectedness of the network structure, making it difficult for emotions to be spread. However, social media platforms do not seem to have an incentive to do so: reducing these posts containing radical statements and emotions would mean a decrease in online social engagement [45]. Therefore, it would be more effective for the entire social platform industry to reach a consensus in this regard. Second, individual characteristics differ in discriminating information and emotions [57], and in general, education is inversely related to online social expression [58]. More educated people care about the content of information when they are exposed to it rather than the subjective emotions of others. This requires governments or institutions to make science knowledge available to the public as much as possible. In addition, the Positive Netizen Strategy seems to be more harmless than the Government Strategy: the Positive Netizen Strategy does not cause an increase in negative emotions, suggesting that improving the quality of individuals and discouraging malicious manipulation of emotions may be a more socially beneficial initiative. Finally, differences in disaster environments may induce different negative public sentiment events. Under an epidemic, negative events expose problems in epidemic preparedness and people focus more on solving existing problems rather than ignoring them. While the mitigation of an epidemic has a significant effect on overall human health, it does not address the specific problems revealed by the negative events. Therefore, additional staffing is needed to specifically address existing problems while ensuring the smooth operation of the epidemic prevention efforts.

5. Conclusions

We construct a model of public sentiment transmission under an epidemic based on theories such as system dynamics and cross-validation, and propose a framework that can be used to improve the model. By analyzing the mechanism and influencing factors of online public sentiment dissemination, a specific SD model is constructed to simulate the dissemination process of public sentiment system. Finally, the validity and rationality of the model are proved through real classical cases. On this basis, the in-fluence of governmental behavior, netizens behavior and disaster context on the propagation of public sentiment is analyzed, and a series of conclusions are drawn: (1) increased government response facilitates the spread of positive sentiment; (2) positive individual behavior contributes to an increase in positive sentiment; (3) changes in the disaster environment (epidemic) affect the spread of sentiment, but the effect is mediocre.

This paper provides a new idea for modeling the public sentiment system under sudden disasters, and also provides theoretical support for relevant organizations to take measures to guide public sentiment. However, our model only considers the situation where the government actively deals with negative events. We suggest that future research could be based on this study by including different governmental attitudes in the model and conducting a precise sentiment analysis of the data, which might lead to more interesting and meaningful results.

Author Contributions: Conceptualization, H.H. and T.X.; Methodology, H.H. and T.X.; Writing—original draft, H.H. and T.X.; Writing—review & editing, W.C., W.W., Y.W.; software, H.H. and Z.F.; visualization, H.H. and Z.F.; supervision, W.C. and W.W.; funding acquisition, T.X. and Y.W. All authors have read and agreed to the published version of the manuscript.

Funding: The paper is supported by National Natural Science Foundation of China (No. 71974090); Natural Science Foundation of Hunan Province of China (No. 2018JJ2336); Philosophy and Social Science Foundation of Hunan Province of China (18YBQ105); Youth talents support program of Hunan Province of China (2018HXQ03); Key scientific research project of Education Department(No. 20A443); Social Science Key Breeding Project of USC (2018XZX16); Doctoral scientific research foundation of USC (No. 2013XQD27); Philosophy and Social Science Foundation Youth Project of Hunan Province of China (19YBQ093); Scientific research project of Education Department (No. 20C1625);and the research is also supported by the "Double Tops" Discipline of Management Science and Engineering of USC.

Informed Consent Statement: Not applicable.

Data Availability Statement: Data available in a publicly accessible repository that does not issue DOIs. Publicly available datasets were analyzed in this study. This data can be found here: https://s.weibo.com/ and https://ef.zhiweidata.com/library.

Acknowledgments: Thanks to Krista Chen for the paper writing advice.

Conflicts of Interest: The authors declare no conflict of interest.

Appendix A

Algorithm A1. Reverse Regression

Input: Dependent variables data y, other independent variables data *othervar*, the number of iterations NI, initial share factor data *sharefactor*, the number of iterations NRI, Maximum and minimum values assumed for *sharefactor* variable *mins* and *maxs*.
LD = The number of dependent variables
for i **in** 0 to LD:
for $i2$ **in** 0 to NI:
for $i3$ **in** 0 to NRI:
n = Generate a random number from 0 to the length of *sharefactor* data
for $i4$ **in** *mins* to *maxs*:
Convert the nth value of *sharefactor* to $i4$.
Calculate the goodness-of-fit of the regression of *othervar* and *sharefactor* on the y (Equation (5)).
Obtain the *sharefactor* with the highest $r2$.
Obtain NI *sharefactor* with the highest $r2$.
Obtain the LD * NI matrix of *sharefactor* with the highest $r2$.
SFMATRIX = the LD * NI matrix of *sharefactor* with the highest $r2$

for *i1* **in** 0 to LD:
    for *i2* **in** the *i1*th column of SFMATRIX:
    for *i3* **in** numbers from 0 to LD except *i1*:
    for *i4* **in** the *i3*th column of SFMATRIX:
Calculate the *r2* of *i2* and *i4*
Obtain *i4* with highest r2
Obtain LD—1 *sharefactor* that are most similar to the trend of *i2* in all columns except for column *i1*.
    Each *sharefactor,* in the *i1*th column of SFMATRIX, gets LD—1 *sharefactor* that are most similar to it
Each *sharefactor,* in SFMATRIX, gets LD—1 *sharefactor* that are most similar to it
SIMLARM = LD * NI matrix of *sharefactor* with similar trends among different dependent variables
Choose the most similar trend in SIMLARM.
Output: *Sharefactor* with the most similar trend among different dependent variables

Algorithm A2. Cross-Validation in the Selection of Linear Models

Input: Dependent variables data *y* and independent variables data *id*, deterministic variables DV and uncertain variables UV, the lowest goodness-of-fit (GOF) that can do cross-validation G.
IN = None
while GOF < G:
    RV = UV except IN
    DV = add IN to DV
    for *i* **in** RV:
Linear regression of the DV and *i* on the dependent variable.
Calculate the goodness-of-fit (GOF)
    Select the *i* with the highest GOF.
    IN = *i*
UV = UV except DV
for *i* **in** 0 to the number of UV:
CV = Combine *i* variables from UV
for *i2* **in** CV:
add *i2* to DV.
Separate data by 8:2 as training and validation sets.
Train set train model (liner regression).
Calculate the validation set error (GOF) using the trained model.
Select the model with the highest GOF in the validation set.
Select the model with the highest GOF in the validation set.
Output: The best model with the highest GOF in the validation set.

Table A1. Model equations.

Name	Abbreviation	Equations	Method	Initial Value
Time	T	T = [1,2,3,4,5,6]	-	0
	Explanation: Iteration time of the model			
R Discussions	RD	$\frac{dRD}{dT} = RND$	ODE	0
	Explanation: Level of network discussion after the government response			
P Discussions	PD	$\frac{dPD}{dT} = ND$	ODE	0
	Explanation: Level of network discussion before the government response			
R Government Speed	RGS	Constants: 2	-	-
	Explanation: Speed of government response, measured in days			
Epidemic Factor	EF	EF = 0.4 * (NC − 0)/(3887 − 0) + 0.6 * (NEC − 0)/(58,097 − 0)	Min-Max scaling	0
	Explanation: Weighted sum of the number of new and existing infections			
Now Confirm	NC	Constants: 5691	-	-
	Explanation: Number of new infections			
New Confirm	NEC	Constants: 2644	-	-
	Explanation: Number of current infections			
Sharefactor	SF	Constants: 3.75	Reverse Regression	-
Explanation: Factors that represent constants during the event, such as the nature of the event itself, the education level of netizens, etc.				

Table A1. Cont.

Name	Abbreviation	Equations	Method	Initial Value
Netizen Posts	NP	NP = POISSON (1874.116 * 1 + 4554.442 * GFOC * T + 0.27 * GF * CMR − 364.268 * GFOC * RGR − 714.778 * T + 86.904 * SF − 0.097 * GF * RCMF + 54.022 * T ** 2 − 4298.99 * GFOC − 11.608 * GFOC * CMR + 1666.766 * GFOC * RCMR − 108.324 * GFOC * RCMF − 1.767 * GFOC * RNP − 5.154 * GR + 0.501 * GR * T − 2.272 * BMP − 17.548 * GFOC * GF − 0.034 * RNP * RCMR) Explanation: Number of original postings by netizen	Liner Regression & poisson	0
Commercial Media Posts	CMP	CMP = POISSON (6.022 * 1 + 0.023 * NP * GFOC + 3.065 * SF + 21.104 * GFOC − 29.066 * T + 2.183 * T ** 2 + 15.346 * EF) Explanation: Number of posts in commercial media	Liner Regression & poisson	0
Commercial Media Reposts	CMR	CMR = POISSON (78.17 * 1 − 0.034 * RCMF * RCMR − 76.7 * T + 9.187 * SF + 0.324 * CMF * GFOC − 0.177 * CMF + 17.044 * EF − 2.539 * GFOC * GP + 0.001 * GF ** 2 − 0.032 * NP − 0.0 * NP ** 2 + 0.035 * GF * RCMF − 0.002 * GF * RNP − 0.017 * NP * RCMF + 0.004 * CMF * RNP + 0.154 * RNP + 0.032 * NP * T − 0.061 * NP * RCMR + 0.001 * NP * RGR + 0.001 * CMF * NP − 0.011 * CMF ** 2 + 5.016 * T ** 2 + 0.293 * CMF * RCMR + 0.003 * GP * RNP − 0.132 * GP * RCMF + 1.939 * GFOC * RGR − 41.531 * GFOC − 3.366 * GR + 1.197 * BMP − 0.001 * GF * BMP − 0.31 * BMP * T + 17.044 * EF) Explanation: Number of commercial media posts retweeted	Liner Regression & poisson	0
Commercial Media Followers	CMF	CMF = 65.935 * 1 − 20.438 * T + 0.416 * SF + 1.441 * T ** 2 + 0.477 * GFOC ** 2 + 0.021 * RCMR * T + 0.0 * GF ** 2 + 0.0 * RCMP * NP + 0.021 * GR * T + 0.024 * RCMP * T − 0.0 * RNP * RCMR − 0.288 * GP * T + 0.097 * GFOC * BMP + 0.023 * NP * T − 0.034 * NP − 0.0 * NP * BMP + 0.037 * GF*RCMR + 0.002 * GFOC * NP − 0.781 * RCMF − 0.037 * GFOC * RCMF + 0.8 * GFOC * T + 0.133 * RCMF * T + 0.002 * RCMF * NP − 0.656 * GFOC * GP + 1.863 * GFOC * RCMR + 0.0 * GP * RNP − 0.029 * GR * RCMR + 0.783 * EF Explanation: The average number of followers of commercial media involved in the event discussion, indicating the influence of commercial media	Liner Regression	0
Commercial Media Discussions	CMD	CMD = CMP * CMR Explanation: The sum of netizens discussions within commercial media	-	0
Government Posts	GP	GP = POISSON (20.262 * 1 − 1.483 * GFOC ** 2 − 1.384 * SF − 0.0 * BMP ** 2 + 13.428 * GFOC + 0.0 * NP * BMP + 0.215 * GFOC * BMP − 0.344 * BMP − 0.042 * NP * GFOC + 0.254 * BMP * T + −4.084 * EF) Explanation: Number of government media postings	Liner Regression & poisson	0
Government Reposts	GR	GR = POISSON (3.462 * 1 + 0.0 * BMP ** 2 − 1.232 * SF + 2.917 * GFOC ** 2 − 0.038 * GF * GFOC + 0.0 * NP ** 2 + 0.001 * GF * RCMF + 0.0 * GF * NP + 0.003 * BMP * RCMF − 0.028 * BMP * T + 0.317 * EF) Explanation: Number of government media posts retweeted	Liner Regression & poisson	0
Government Followers	GF	GF = 102.26 * 1 + 0.191 * GFOC * RNP + −9.552 * SF + 0.007 * CMR * BMP + −13.49 * T + 0.64 * T ** 2 + −0.073 * BMP * RGR + 0.001 * RGR ** 2 + −0.02 * GFOC * NP + 0.107 * GFOC * BMP + −0.003 * NP * RCMF + −1.624 * GFOC * RCMF + −0.002 * CMR * RCMF + 0.056 * RCMF * T + 0.011 * RCMF * RGR + −0.028 * RCMR ** 2 + 0.112 * RCMR * T + 1.078 * RCMR + 1.987 * GFOC * RGR + 3.286 * GFOC * RCMR + 0.012 * CMR * RCMR + 0.0 * NP * BMP + −0.45 * RNP + −0.0 * RCMP ** 2 + 0.015 * BMP * RCMP + 0.002 * RNP * RCMF Explanation: The average number of followers of government media involved in the event discussion, indicating the influence of government media	Liner Regression	0
Government Discussions	GD	GD = GP * GR Explanation: The sum of netizen discussions within government media	-	0
Network Discussions	ND	ND = NP+ BMD + GD Explanation: Total postings by netizens, government and commercial media before government response	-	0
R Netizen Posts	RNP	RNP = POISSON (−298.162 * 1 + 4.712 * BMP + 10.359 * SF − 0.007 * RGP * BMP − 0.017 * RGR * CMR + 3.092 * RGP * T + 0.019 * GP * GR + 56.422 * EF) Explanation: The number of original posts from netizens after the government response.	Liner Regression & poisson	0
R Commercial Media Posts	RCMP	RCMP = POISSON (−67.288 * 1 + 2.357 * RGP + 1.491 * SF − 0.071 * CMR * GP + 0.432 * GFOC * GF − 0.053 * RGR * RGP + 0.079 * RGR * GP + 0.063 * RGP * CMR + 14.523 * EF) Explanation: Number of commercial media postings after government response	Liner Regression & poisson	0

Table A1. Cont.

Name	Abbreviation	Equations	Method	Initial Value
R Commercial Media Reposts	RCMR	RCMR = POISSON (−4.361 * 1 + 0.006 * RCMF * RGR + 1.129 * SF − 0.001 * RGR ** 2 + 0.013 * CMR + 0.02 * GP + 0.007 * RCMF * T − 0.041 * BMP − 0.001 * CMR * BMP + 0.046 * BMP * T − 0.0 * NP * GR)	Liner Regression & poisson	0
Explanation: Retweeted commercial media posts after government response				
R Commercial Media Followers	RCMF	RCMF = 127.299 * 1 − 0.924 * RGF + 2.676 * SF − 43.353 * T − 0.084 * CMR * GR + 0.0 * NP * GR + 0.014 * GP * GR + 0.011 * CMR * GF + 2.827 * T ** 2 + 0.157 * RGF * T − 0.245 * GF * T − 0.025 * RGR * GP + 2.698 * EF + 2.981 * GR * T + 0.003 * RGF * GR + 0.306 * GP * T + 0.29 * GFOC * RGF − 0.06 * RGR * GR − 0.089 * NP − 0.138 * GFOC * RGP + 0.007 * RGR * RGF + 2.698 * EF	Liner Regression	0
Explanation: The average followers of commercial media involved in the discussion of the event after the government response				
R Commercial Media Discussions	RCMD	RCMD = RCMP * RCMR	-	0
Explanation: Total netizen discussion within the commercial media after the government response				
R Government Posts	RGP	RGP = POISSON ([0,305,3,0,0,0])	real data & poisson	0
Explanation: Number of government response postings after the government response				
R Government Reposts	RGR	RGR = POISSON (−23.102 * 1 − 0.0 * NP ** 2 + 3.439 * SF − 0.093 * BMP * T + 0.002 * RGF * CMR − 0.391 * GR * T − 0.0 * RGF ** 2 − 0.001 * GF ** 2 + 0.002 * RGF * GF + 0.002 * CMR * NP + 0.004 * BMP * GR + 0.174 * RGF − 26.594 * GFOC + 0.054 * NP − 0.0 * CMR ** 2 + 2.363 * EF)	Liner Regression & poisson	0
Explanation: Number of government media postings retweeted by netizens after government response				
R Government Followers	RGF	RGF = [0,444,158,0,0,0]	Real Data	0
Explanation: Average number of government media followers after government response				
R Government Discussions	RGD	RGD = RGP * RGR	-	0
Explanation: Total network discussions within government media after government response				
R Network Discussions	RND	RND = RNP + RBMD + RGD	-	0
Explanation: Total postings and reposts by netizens, government and commercial media after the government response				
Government Focus	GFOC	GFOC = (RGP * RGF − 0)/(253,132 − 0) * 10	Min-Max scaling	0
Explanation: The level of government media involvement in the event discussion.				
Public Sentiment	PS	PS = RD − PD	-	0
Explanation: Propagation of public sentiment before and after the response				

Note: * is for multiplication and ** is for power operations.

References

1. COVID-19 Weekly Epidemiological Update. Available online: https://www.who.int/publications/m/item/weekly-epidemiological-update---29-december-2020 (accessed on 30 December 2020).
2. Kiecolt-Glaser, J.K.; McGuire, L.; Robles, T.F.; Glaser, R. Emotions, morbidity, and mortality: New perspectives from psychoneuroimmunology. *Annu. Rev. Psychol.* **2002**, *53*, 83–107. [CrossRef] [PubMed]
3. Schaller, M.; Murray, D.R.; Bangerter, A. Implications of the behavioral immune system for social behavior and human health in the modern world. *Philos. Trans. Biol. Sci.* **2015**, *370*, 1–10. [CrossRef]
4. Kalichman, S. Denying AIDS: Conspiracy theories, pseudoscience, and human tragedy. *Afr. Aff.* **2009**, *109*, 505–506. [CrossRef]
5. Farmer, P. *AIDS and Accusation: Haiti and the Geography of Blame*, 1st ed.; University of California Press: Berkeley, CA, USA, 2006; p. 372.
6. Bogart, L.M.; Wagner, G.; Galvan, F.H.; Banks, D. Conspiracy beliefs about HIV are related to antiretroviral treatment: Nonadherence among African American men with HIV. *J. Acquir. Immune. Defic. Syndr.* **2010**, *53*, 648–655. [CrossRef] [PubMed]
7. Gilles, I.; Bangerter, A.; Clémence, A.; Green, E.G.T.; Krings, F.; Staerklé, C.; Wagner-Egger, P. Trust in medical organizations predicts pandemic (H1N1) 2009 vaccination behavior and perceived efficacy of protection measures in the Swiss public. *Eur. J. Epidemiol.* **2011**, *26*, 203–210. [CrossRef] [PubMed]
8. DeStefano, F.; Shimabukuro, T.T. The MMR vaccine and autism. *Annu. Rev. Virol.* **2019**, *6*, 585–600. [CrossRef] [PubMed]
9. Hills, P.; Argyle, M. The oxford happiness questionnaire: A compact scale for the measurement of psychological well-being. *Pers. Individ. Differ.* **2002**, *33*, 1073–1082. [CrossRef]
10. Derogatis, L.R.; Lipman, R.S.; Covi, L. SCL-90: An outpatient psychiatric rating scale–Preliminary report. *Psychopharmacol. Bull.* **1973**, *9*, 13–28. [PubMed]
11. Larsen, K.S.; Cary, W.; Chaplin, B.; Deane, D.; Green, R.; Hyde, W.; Zuleger, K. Women's liberation: The development of a likert-type scale. *J. Soc. Psychol.* **1976**, *98*, 295–296. [CrossRef]
12. Hong, Y.; Lee, T.; Kim, J.S. Serial Multiple Mediation Analyses: How to Enhance Individual Public Health Emergency Preparedness and Response to Environmental Disasters. *Int. J. Environ. Res. Public Health* **2019**, *16*, 223. [CrossRef]

13. Li, S.; Wang, Y.; Xue, J.; Zhao, N.; Zhu, T. The Impact of COVID-19 Epidemic Declaration on Psychological Consequences: A Study on Active Weibo Users. *Int. J. Environ. Res. Public Health* **2020**, *17*, 2032. [CrossRef]
14. Apuke, O.D.; Omar, B. Fake News and COVID-19: Modelling the Predictors of Fake News Sharing Among Social Media Users. *Telemat. Inform.* **2020**, *56*, 101475. [CrossRef]
15. Hong, Y.; Zhang, P. Political news and happiness: The difference between traditional media and new media use. *Chin. J. Commun.* **2020**, *13*, 370–388. [CrossRef]
16. Liu, D.; Wang, W.; Li, H. Evolutionary Mechanism and Information Supervision of Public Opinions in Internet Emergency. *Procedia Comput. Sci.* **2013**, *17*, 973–980. [CrossRef]
17. Naskar, D.; Singh, S.; Kumar, D.; Nandi, S.; Rivaherrera, E. Emotion Dynamics of Public Opinions on Twitter. *ACM Trans. Inf. Syst.* **2020**, *38*, 18. [CrossRef]
18. Xie, T.; Wei, Y.; Chen, W.; Huang, H. Parallel evolution and response decision method for public sentiment based on system dynamics. *Eur. J. Oper. Res.* **2020**, *287*, 1131–1148. [CrossRef] [PubMed]
19. Sun, W.; Zhao, C.; Wang, Y.; Cho, C.H. Corporate social responsibility disclosure and catering to investor sentiment in China. *Manag. Decis.* **2018**, *56*, 1917–1935. [CrossRef]
20. Danso, A.; Lartey, T.; Amankwah-Amoah, J.; Adomako, S.; Lu, Q.; Uddin, M. Market sentiment and firm investment decision-making. *Int. Rev. Financ. Anal.* **2019**, *66*, 101369. [CrossRef]
21. Geisser, S. A Predictive Approach to the Random Effect Model. *Biometrika* **1974**, *61*, 101–107. [CrossRef]
22. Devroye, L.; Wagner, T.J. Distribution-Free performance bounds for potential function rules. *IEEE Trans. Inf. Theory* **1979**, *25*, 601–604. [CrossRef]
23. Bañuls, V.A.; Turoff, M.; Roxanne, S. Collaborative scenario modeling in emergency management through cross-impact. *Technol. Forecast. Soc. Chang.* **2013**, *80*, 1756–1774. [CrossRef]
24. Davis, J.P.; Eisenhardt, K.M.; Bingham, C.B. Developing theory through simulation methods. *Acad. Manag. Rev.* **2007**, *32*, 480–499. [CrossRef]
25. Rogers, G.; Chow, J. Hands-on teaching of power system dynamics. *IEEE Comput. Appl. Power* **1995**, *8*, 12–16. [CrossRef]
26. Mcquail, D.; Windahl, S. *Communication Models for the Study of Mass Communications*, 2nd ed.; Routledge: Oxford, UK, 1981; pp. 138–140.
27. Sterman, J. System dynamics modelling: Tools for learning in a complex world. *Calif. Manag. Rev.* **2001**, *43*, 8–25. [CrossRef]
28. Rahmandada, H.; Sterman, J.D. Reporting guidelines for simulation-based research in social sciences. *Syst. Dyn. Rev.* **2012**, *28*, 396–411. [CrossRef]
29. Weibo Search Weibo Topic. Available online: https://s.weibo.com/ (accessed on 1 May 2020).
30. Che, X.H.; Ip, B. *Social Networks in China*, 1st ed.; Chandos: Cambridge, MA, USA, 2018; pp. 87–100.
31. Tencent WeChat Subscriptions Platform. Available online: https://mp.weixin.qq.com/ (accessed on 1 May 2020).
32. Zhiweidata Events Library. Available online: https://ef.zhiweidata.com/library (accessed on 1 May 2020).
33. Huo, L.; Huang, P.; Fang, X. An interplay model for authorities' actions and rumor spreading in emergency event. *Phys. A Stat. Mech. Appl.* **2011**, *390*, 3267–3274. [CrossRef]
34. Briones, R.L.; Kuch, B.; Liu, B.F.; Jin, Y. Keeping up with the digital age: How the American Red Cross uses social media to build relationships. *Public Relat. Rev.* **2011**, *37*, 37–43. [CrossRef]
35. Coombs, W.T. Protecting Organization Reputations During a Crisis: The Development and Application of Situational Crisis Communication Theory. *Corp. Reput. Rev.* **2007**, *10*, 163–176. [CrossRef]
36. Huffaker, D. Dimensions of Leadership and Social Influence in Online Communities. *Hum. Commun. Res.* **2010**, *36*, 593–617. [CrossRef]
37. Yu, L.; Li, L.; Tang, L. What can mass media do to control public panic in accidents of hazardous chemical leakage into rivers? A multi-agent-based online opinion dissemination model. *J. Clean. Prod.* **2017**, *143*, 1203–1214. [CrossRef]
38. Dyda, A.; Shah, Z.; Surian, D.; Martin, P.; Coiera, E.; Dey, A.; Leask, J.; Dunn, A.G. HPV vaccine coverage in Australia and associations with HPV vaccine information exposure among Australian Twitter users. *Hum. Vaccines Immunother.* **2019**, *15*, 1488–1495. [CrossRef] [PubMed]
39. Blanchard-Boehm, R.D.; Cook, M.J. Risk Communication and Public Education in Edmonton, Alberta, Canada on the 10th Anniversary of the "Black Friday" Tornado. *Int. Res. Geogr. Environ. Educ.* **2004**, *13*, 38–54. [CrossRef]
40. Balathé, M.; Vu, D.Q.; Khandelwal, S.; Hunter, D.R. The dynamics of health behavior sentiments on a large online social network. *EPJ Data Sci.* **2013**, *2*, 4. [CrossRef]
41. Rosenbusch, H.; Evans, A.M.; Zeelenberg, M. Multilevel Emotion Transfer on YouTube: Disentangling the Effects of Emotional Contagion and Homophily on Video Audiences. *Soc. Psychol. Personal. Sci.* **2019**, *10*, 1028–1035. [CrossRef]
42. Fowler, J.H.; Christakis, N.A. Dynamic spread of happiness in a large social network: Longitudinal analysis over 20 years in the Framingham Heart Study. *BMJ* **2008**, *337*, a2338. [CrossRef]
43. Goldenberg, A.; Gross, J.J. Digital Emotion Contagion. *Trends Cogn. Sci.* **2020**, *24*, 316–328. [CrossRef] [PubMed]
44. Kramer, A.D.I. The spread of emotion via facebook. *Assoc. Comput. Mach.* **2012**, 767–770. [CrossRef]
45. Kramer, A.D.I.; Guillory, J.E.; Hancock, J.T. Experimental evidence of massivescale emotional contagion through social networks. *Proc. Natl. Acad. Sci. USA* **2014**, *111*, 8788–8790. [CrossRef] [PubMed]

46. Xiong, X.; Li, Y.; Qiao, S.; Han, N.; Wu, Y.; Peng, J.; Li, B. An emotional contagion model for heterogeneous social media with multiple behaviors. *Phys. A Stat. Mech. Its Appl.* **2018**, *490*, 185–202. [CrossRef]
47. Zhao, L.; Cheng, J.; Qian, Y.; Wang, Q. USEIRS model for the contagion of individual aggressive behavior under emergencies. *Simulation* **2012**, *88*, 1456–1464. [CrossRef]
48. Ferrara, E.; Yang, Z. Measuring emotional contagion in social media. *PLoS ONE* **2015**, *10*, e0142390. [CrossRef] [PubMed]
49. Del Vicario, M.; Vivaldo, G.; Bessi, A.; Zollo, F.; Scala, A.; Caldarelli, G.; Quattrociocchi, W. Echo Chambers: Emotional Contagion and Group Polarization on Facebook. *Sci. Rep.* **2016**, *6*, 1–12. [CrossRef] [PubMed]
50. Diaz, A.; Eisenberg, N. The Process of Emotion Regulation Is Different From Individual Differences in Emotion Regulation: Conceptual Arguments and a Focus on Individual Differences. *Psychol. Inq.* **2015**, *26*, 37–47. [CrossRef]
51. Eachempati, P.; Srivastava, P.R.; Zhang, Z.J. Gauging opinions about the COVID-19: A multi-channel social media approach. *Enterp. Inf. Syst.* **2020**, 1–35. [CrossRef]
52. Zhu, B.; Zheng, X.; Liu, H.; Li, J.; Wang, P. Analysis of spatiotemporal characteristics of big data on social media sentiment with COVID-19 epidemic topics. *Chaos Solitons Fractals* **2020**, *140*, 110123. [CrossRef] [PubMed]
53. Li, Q.; Wei, C.; Dang, J.; Cao, L.; Liu, L. Tracking and Analyzing Public Emotion Evolutions During COVID-19: A Case Study from the Event-Driven Perspective on Microblogs. *Int. J. Environ. Res. Public Health* **2020**, *17*, 6888. [CrossRef]
54. Bertot, J.C.; Jaeger, P.T.; Grimes, J.M. Using ICTs to create a culture of transparency: E-government and social media as openness and anti-corruption tools for societies. *Gov. Inf. Q.* **2010**, *27*, 264–271. [CrossRef]
55. Jung, J.-Y.; Moro, M. Multi-level functionality of social media in the aftermath of the Great East Japan Earthquake. *Disasters* **2014**, *38*, s123–s143. [CrossRef] [PubMed]
56. Branicki, L.J.; Agyei, D.A. Unpacking the Impacts of Social Media Upon Crisis Communication and City Evacuation. In *City Evacuations: An Interdisciplinary Approach*; Springer: Berlin, Germany, 2015; pp. 21–37. [CrossRef]
57. Hong, Y.; Kim, J.-S.; Xiong, L. Media Exposure and Individuals' Emergency Preparedness Behaviors for Coping with Natural and Human-Made Disasters. *J. Environ. Psychol.* **2019**, *63*, 82–91. [CrossRef]
58. Stokes, C.; Senkbeil, J.C. Facebook and Twitter, communication and shelter, and the 2011 Tuscaloosa tornado. *Disasters* **2016**, *41*, 194–208. [CrossRef]

International Journal of
Environmental Research and Public Health

Article

Place Attachment and Household Disaster Preparedness: Examining the Mediation Role of Self-Efficacy

Ziyi Wang [1], Ziqiang Han [1], Lin Liu [1,2] and Shaobin Yu [1,*]

[1] School of Political Science and Public Administration, Shandong University, Qingdao 266237, China; ziyi.wang.em@mail.sdu.edu.cn (Z.W.); ziqiang.han@sdu.edu.cn (Z.H.); liulinsdu@sdu.edu.cn (L.L.)
[2] Institute of Governance, Shandong University, Qingdao 266237, China
* Correspondence: shaobinyu@sdu.edu.cn

Abstract: Household preparedness is essential for resilience-building and disaster risk reduction. Limited studies have explored the correlations between place attachment, self-efficacy, and disaster preparedness, especially in the east Asian cultural context. This study investigates the mediating role of self-efficacy between place attachment and disaster preparedness based on data from the 2018 Shandong General Social Survey (N = 2181) in China. We categorized the preparedness behaviors into three specific clusters: material, behavioral and awareness preparedness. Multiple linear regressions and the Sobel Goodman tests were employed to estimate the correlations with the control of necessary confounding variables such as disaster experience, socioeconomic and demographic characteristics. The results demonstrate that both the place attachment and self-efficacy are correlated with higher degrees of overall preparedness and all three types of preparedness, and self-efficacy plays a mediating role between place attachment and disaster preparedness. These findings highlight the importance of promoting place attachment and self-efficacy in the advocacies and outreach activities of disaster preparedness.

Keywords: place attachment; self-efficacy; disaster preparedness; disaster experience; China

1. Introduction

Disaster preparedness, as the knowledge and capacities developed by institutions, communities, and individuals to anticipate, respond to, and recover from the impacts of all disasters and the related efforts of increasing such knowledge and capacities [1], is essential to reduce the impact of a disaster. Pre-disaster risk reduction efforts include both mitigation and preparedness activities. Some scholars and practitioners differentiate the two concepts. They suggest that mitigation activities are related to the physical and engineering efforts and long-run solutions (e.g., building sea walls) [2,3], while the preparedness activities are more about the knowledge and capacity building activities, but some other researchers treat all the pre-event mitigation and preparedness activities as similar concepts [4,5]. Disaster preparedness behaviors include all the actions taken to reduce the potential impact of potential disasters. In general, disaster activities can be divided into material preparedness (e.g., preparing an emergency kit at home), awareness or knowledge preparedness (e.g., learning knowledge about disasters), and behavioral preparedness (e.g., participating in exercise or drills, being a volunteer) [6,7], and during the emergent situation, information seeking, emotional coping, and the adoption of protective actions (e.g., emergency evacuation) are the general clusters of preparedness behaviors [8]. Regarding the entities of disaster preparedness, they can be implemented either by individuals/households or organizations such as government agencies [9–11] or business companies [12]. Previous calculation using data from the United States of America indicated that one dollar of investment in pre-disaster mitigation and preparedness efforts could prevent six dollars in losses from potential disasters [13]. Since the "whole community" approach is suggested and all stakeholders are encouraged to engage in disaster preparedness [14], the disaster preparedness of individuals and households, which are the basic social unit and the very frontline of disaster response, deserve to be further investigated.

Scholars have developed or adopted various theoretical frameworks to understand the predictors and barriers of preparedness behaviors in the face of risk, such as the protective action decision model, health belief model, extended parallel process model, theory of planned behavior, social cognitive theories, and personal-relative-to-event model, etc., and all these frameworks were concentrated in the social-psychological and behavioral science domain [6,15]. The social-cognitive framework highlights the importance of place attachment, types of efficacy, and perceived responsibility among stakeholders in predicting the adoption of preparedness behaviors, but the effects of these variables in individual and household disaster preparedness are insufficiently investigated in empirical studies [15,16]. Therefore, inspired by the social cognitive framework in disaster studies [16], we developed this study by investigating the complex relationships between place attachment, self-efficacy, and disaster preparedness behaviors.

Place attachment refers to the affect and emotions that connect people to places or physical environment [17,18]. It can influence an individual's intention to prepare or the actual preparedness behaviors, especially in times of stress. Place attachment is a crucial concept widely used in environmental studies and adopted in cross-disciplinary natural hazards research. However, the effects of place attachment on risk perception and disaster preparedness varied in different cultural and hazard contexts in current studies. Bonaiuto's review of 31 studies investigating the correlations between place attachment and natural hazards risk perceptions found that there were both positive and negative relations between place attachment and risk perception, place attachment, and risk coping behaviors [19]. Moreover, place attachment can affect the risk perception and coping behaviors in multiple ways, either directly or indirectly, as moderating or mediating roles [18–20].

Place attachment can drive individuals' personal emotions into practical actions that protect themselves and their communities [20]. This assumption was supported in India regarding flood preparedness [18] and in southwest China regarding insurance purchasing intention toward landslides [21]. Nevertheless, a more substantial place attachment may lead to underestimating potential risks [22,23], or unwillingness to relocate, or a greater likelihood of returning to risky areas after a natural disaster [19,24]. The effect of place attachment on individuals' risk perceptions and risk coping behaviors can be mediated by variables such as longevity in or the familiarity with a place [25]. It can also be moderated by variables such as the environmental contexts or the types of attachments. For example, in a study about wildfire mitigation and preparedness in Australia, place attachment can only motivate the residents' preparedness actions in the rural sample, but not in the urban and the wildland–urban interface samples [26]. A similar study about flood preparedness in Orissa, India, also revealed that although genealogical and economical attachment to a place contributed to flood preparedness, religious attachment did not [18].

Self-efficacy is considered as an individual's belief or perception about his/her capacity to practice or implement a task or action [27]. Generally, collective efficacy, response/outcome efficacy are similar efficacy concepts used in literature along with self-efficacy. The response efficacy [28], also termed as outcome efficacy [29,30], refers to the belief or perception of the usefulness or effectiveness of the protective activities or the adaptative behaviors. Similarly, collective efficacy refers to the belief or perception of a group's conjoint capabilities to organize or do something [31,32]. In the field of disaster research, self-efficacy refers to the assessment of one's own ability to initiate or complete a preventive, protective, or adaptive behavior [29]. Self-efficacy is an essential social cognitive precursor to prepare for disasters in the social-cognitive theory model [16]. People will develop intentions to prepare for disasters only if they have adequate expectations about being able to perform the act [33]. Most studies have demonstrated that high self-efficacy can motivate disaster preparedness intentions or the actual behaviors [30,34,35], or the specific protective actions in emergencies such as emergency evacuation [29]. Such positive effects were primarily observed in preparation for floods [36–39], earthquakes [40], or climate change-related hazards [30]. In household disaster preparedness studies, self-efficacy is always captured by the self-reported confidence of their capacity for implementing a protective action against a disaster or successfully coping with potential disasters [33,39]. It appears that the role of self-efficacy in disaster preparedness is still relatively understudied in terms of geographical, social and cultural diversity, though there is an increasing trend in recent years [30].

The correlation between place attachment and self-efficacy has also been examined a limited amount in the context of disaster risk perception and preparedness studies, because most of the studies have not yet linked the two together. According to the place identity theory, place attachment can produce a stronger sense of self-efficacy [41] because the environment maintains the feeling of self-efficacy facilitation [42]. The familiarity and attachment to a place may make people feel unique, in control of, and good about themselves [43], which eventually provides feelings of distinctiveness, continuity, self-esteem, and self-efficacy [44].

Therefore, guided by the social-cognitive theory, this study aims to investigate the correlations between place attachment, self-efficacy, and household preparedness using a representative survey conducted in 2018 in Shandong province, China. This study can enrich the current knowledge by (1) linking the place attachment, self-efficacy, and disaster preparedness in one model, and exploring their complex relations, as shown in Figure 1; (2) testing these relationships in the context of a place with fewer disasters before but facing increasing threats from climate-related disasters. Furthermore, the findings of this research can improve the social cognitive theory in disaster preparedness studies and eventually promote the individual and household's disaster preparedness activities by promoting their confidence in protecting themselves (efficacy) from potential disasters. Based on the discussions above, we assume that self-efficacy can play a mediating role between place attachment and preparedness; thus, we hypothesize that:

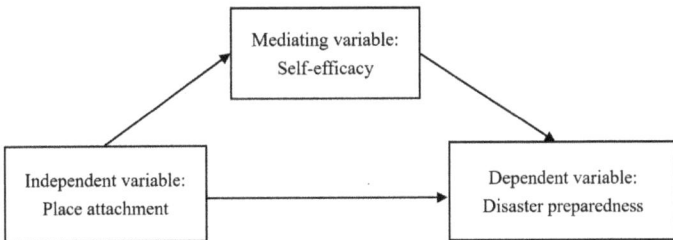

Figure 1. The proposed conceptual model.

Hypothesis 1 (H1). *Place attachment is positively correlated with household preparedness.*

Hypothesis 2 (H2). *A higher degree of self-efficacy predicts a higher degree of preparedness.*

Hypothesis 3 (H3). *Self-efficacy mediates the relationship between place attachment and disaster preparedness.*

2. Methods

2.1. Study Area and Participants

Data used in this analysis comes from a representative survey from Shandong province. As a coastal province of China, Shandong severely suffered from flood risk about 100 years ago due to the unstable situation of the Huang River [45]. However, during the decades after the establishment of the People's Republic of China in 1949, the province has experienced much fewer occurrences of natural-induced disasters [46]. Nevertheless, more and more typhoons have hit this area in recent years. In 2018, the typhoon Rumbia hit

Shandong province, followed by another typhoon, Lekima, in 2019 [47–49], as shown in Figure 2a,b. Typhoon Rumbia affected more than 1.47 million residents and caused a direct economic loss of about 9.2 billion Chinese Yuan (about 1.3 billion US dollars) [50]. Likewise, typhoon Lekima affected more than 1.66 million residents; among them, 183,800 had to be evacuated. It was estimated that direct economic loss was about 1.5 billion Chinese Yuan (about USD $212 million) due to the collapse of houses and the losses of agricultural productions [51]. In this scenario, studies about residents' preparedness behaviors based on data from Shandong province are precious because the public has not experienced disasters for quite a long time, but the prospect of disasters looms large, especially typhoons and related floods.

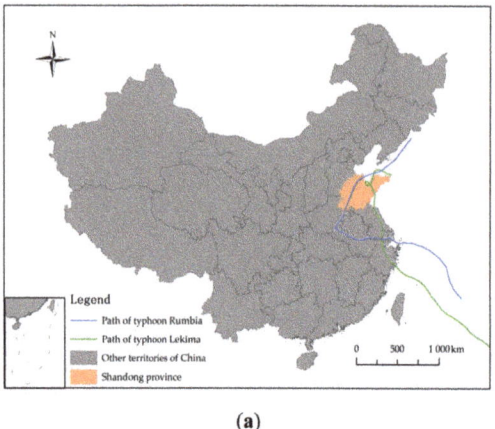 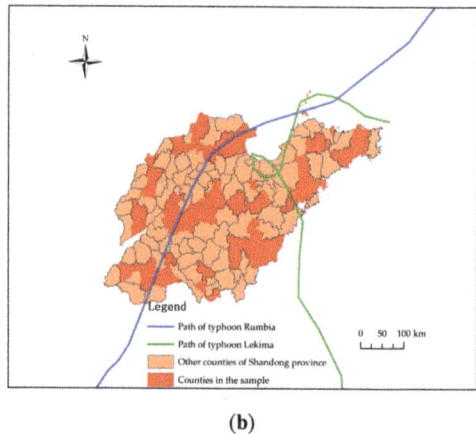

(a) (b)

Figure 2. (a) The location of Shandong province and paths of Typhoon Rumbia and Lekima; (b) Sampled counties in Shandong province and paths of Typhoon Rumbia and Lekima. Note: Data source of typhoon path is from China Meteorological Administration tropical cyclone database. This figure was prepared with ArcGIS 10.7 (ESRI, Redlands, CA, USA).

The Shandong General Social Survey (SGSS) is a large-scale household survey project conducted by Shandong University, and the disaster preparedness module was included in the 2018 survey. The survey used a PPS (probability proportionate to size sampling) sampling strategy, a stratified, four-stage nonprobability sampling method. The primary sampling unit was the county, the second was the town, and the third was communities. Households were then randomly selected within the community using the household registration list. Residents aged 18 and above were the targeted population. We recruited 7382 households, and 4259 individuals in 4259 households responded to our survey, indicating a response rate of 57.69%. Since the disaster preparedness module was only included in one of the two versions of the questionnaire, this data included 2181 participants from 2181 households. Data collection was conducted through face-to-face interviews by trained college students between 26 May 2018 and 9 October 2018, with the assistance of the computer-assisted personal interviewing (CAPI) system. Finally, 1863 valid observations were included in our analysis after the dropping of records with missing values.

2.2. Measures

2.2.1. Disaster Preparedness

Based on prior studies [6,7,52], 18 questions about disaster preparedness activities were incorporated into the survey. Specifically, seven of the questions were related to material preparedness (food, water, flashlight, emergency kit, radio, medicine, special needs) within a household, another seven about their planning and actions linked to disaster risk reduction (behavioral preparedness), and the last four about the participant's awareness of disaster protective actions (awareness preparedness). The seven types of behavioral preparedness activities were "developing a written family emergency plan", "having a reunion plan within family members for potential emergencies", "paying attention to disasters related information", "purchasing accident insurance for family members", "participating in emergency training", "discussing with friends and family members about what to do if emergencies happened", and "being a volunteer or a member of community emergency response team". The four awareness preparedness activities were aware of "how to ask friends and family members for help", "know which government agency to call for help", "know the nearest emergency shelter", and "know the emergency exit."

2.2.2. Place Attachment

The place attachment was estimated by the degree of agreement to two statements: (1) "I have a sense of belonging to our community", and (2) "I am very proud to tell others where I live." The answers to each question ranged from one to five, indicating an increased degree of agreement to the statements. The mean value of the answers to the two questions was used to measure place attachment in this analysis.

2.2.3. Self-Efficacy

Self-efficacy, also termed as one's confidence about one's ability to effectively engage in a behavior [33], can lead to the intention and actual perform of a disaster preparedness behavior [16]. Based on previous literature [33], we measured self-efficacy by the evaluation of the question "how do you evaluate your confidence in yourself or your family's capacity of response if some emergency happens?", and a five-point Likert scale measured the answers from 1 (not confident at all) to 5 (very confident) [29].

2.2.4. Control Variables

Disaster experience, socioeconomic, and demographic variables were included in this analysis as the controlled variables. The disaster experience was measured by a question "Have you experienced the following disasters or emergencies in the last 10 years?" and 13 types of disasters such as earthquake, flood, landslide/debris flow, typhoon, low-temperature freezes/blizzards, droughts, water pollution, air pollution/smog, fires, large-scale infectious diseases (e.g., SARS), nuclear accidents, chemical accidents, and crowd trampling were included. The frequency of choice to each type of emergency was calculated as the experience of disasters. Based on previous literature [6,53–58], we controlled the socioeconomic and demographic variables which were potentially correlated to disaster preparedness, such as the participant's age, whether there are children at home (yes = 1), gender (male = 1), ethnicity (Han = 1), community (rural/urban difference) (urban = 1), marital status (married = 1), Communist Party of China (CPC) membership (yes = 1), religion (yes = 1), education level (illiteracy = 0, primary = 1, middle school = 2, high school = 3, college or above = 4), annual household income (in thousand Chinese Yuan (CNY)), property ownership (yes = 1). Being a member of the Chinese Communist Party is always used as an indicator of political status and capability of acquiring resources in the Chinese context [6,57].

2.3. Data Analysis

We first reported the percentages of the participants' preparedness activities and the descriptive statistics of all the variables. After that, we conducted the OLS (ordinary least squares) regressions by treating all the preparedness activities as one overall preparedness indicator and then used the material preparedness, behavioral preparedness, and awareness preparedness as separate preparedness indicators, respectively. The OLS models were used because we treated the dependent variables as continuous variables in this paper. We calculated the Cronbach's alpha test to check the internal consistency for the concepts that included several variables. The mediation effect of self-efficacy between place attachment and preparedness was also tested using the Sobel Goodman test and the three-step test method [59,60]. All the analyses were conducted by the statistical package Stata 16 (StataCorp, College Station, Texas, TX, USA).

3. Results

3.1. Descriptive Analysis

The aggregation of all the 18 preparative activities was treated as the degree of overall preparedness. The sum of the seven material preparedness activities, the four awareness items, and the seven behavioral activities were treated as the degree of material preparedness, behavioral preparedness, and awareness preparedness, respectively [6,7].

As shown in Table 1, the behavioral aspects of disaster preparedness were comparatively low: only 23.99% had insurance coverage for potential emergencies, 15.51% had a reunion plan within family members for a potential emergency, 9.64% had participated in emergency training, 2.76% had been a volunteer, and 1.47% had drafted a family emergency plan. A total of 55.95% knew the nearest emergency shelter, 27.19% knew the emergency exit and how to evacuate safely, 38.59% knew which government agency to call for help during emergencies, and 75.10% knew how to ask friends and family members for help. For the four material preparedness activities, 82.25% of the participants had prepared a three-day supply of water, 59.59% had prepared a three-day supply of food, 64.90% had a flashlight, 9.90% had an emergency kit, 14.63% had a radio with batteries, 70.46% had necessary medicine for family members, and 14.59% had arranged special needs for women, children or elders.

Table 1. Disaster preparedness activities.

Types	Variables	Frequency	Percentage
Material preparedness	Three-day supply of water	1793	82.25
	Three-day supply of food	1299	59.59
	Flashlight	1415	64.91
	Emergency kit	216	9.91
	Radio with batteries	319	14.63
	Necessary medicine for family members	1536	70.46
	Special needs for women, children or elders	318	14.59
Behavioral preparedness	Having a family emergency plan	32	1.47
	Having a reunion plan within family members for potential emergency	338	15.51
	Paying attention to disasters related information	908	41.69
	Purchasing accident insurance for family members	522	23.99
	Participating in emergency training	210	9.64
	Discussing with friends and family members about what to do if emergencies happened	524	24.06
	Being a volunteer or a member of community emergency response team	60	2.76
Awareness preparedness	Knowing the nearest emergency shelter	1217	55.95
	Knowing the emergency exit and how to evacuate safely	592	27.19
	Knowing which government agency to call for help during emergencies	840	38.59
	Knowing how to ask friends and family members for help	1635	75.10

Place attachment had a mean value of 3.72, with a standard deviation of 0.77, and a Cronbach's alpha test result of 0.78. Self-efficacy had a mean value of 4.25, with a standard deviation of 0.87. Disaster experience ranged from 0 to 12, with a mean value of 2.33, and a standard deviation of 1.80 (Table 2).

Table 2. Descriptive statistics of independent variables.

Variables		N	Mean	SD	Min	Max
Place attachment		2172	3.72	0.77	1	5
Self-efficacy		2172	4.25	0.87	1	5
Disaster experience		2169	2.33	1.80	0	12
Age		2181	53.75	16.63	18	99
Annual household income		1863	57,190	136,786	0	4,000,000
		Frequency		Percent		
Property ownership	Yes	1143		52.41		
	No	1038		47.59		
Education	Illiteracy	511		23.44		
	Primary	515		23.62		
	Middle	618		28.35		
	High	285		13.07		
	College+	251		11.51		
Gender	Female	1193		45.30		
	Male	988		54.70		
Ethnicity	Han	2171		99.54		
	Others	10		0.46		
Community	Rural	2073		95.05		
	Urban	108		4.95		
Religion	None	2067		94.77		
	Yes	114		5.23		
Marital status	Not married	471		21.60		
	Married	1710		78.40		
CPC member	Yes	167		7.67		
	No	2011		92.33		
Child(ren) at home	Yes	1991		91.29		
	No	190		8.71		
Total		2181		100		

As shown in Table 2, within the 2181 participants, 54.70% were male, 99.54% were the Han majority, 96.64% were registered as rural *Hukou*, 5.23% had religious beliefs, 78.40% of them were married, 91.29% had at least one child at home, 52.41% possessed their property right, and 7.67% were CPC members. For education degree, 23.44% of the respondents only attended primary school, 28.35% attended middle school or equivalent, 13.07% attended high school or equivalent, and 11.51% had college or above education experience. On average, the participants were 53.75 years old, and their average annual household income was about 57,190 Chinese Yuan (about 8760 US dollars).

3.2. Correlations between Place Attachment, Self-Efficacy, and Preparedness

This study differentiated the overall preparedness into three categories: material preparedness, behavioral preparedness, and awareness preparedness. As shown in Table 3, both self-efficacy and place attachment are correlated to the overall preparedness indicator, as well as the three different preparedness degrees, in terms of material preparedness, awareness preparedness, and behavioral preparedness.

Table 3. Disaster preparedness and influencing factors (full models).

Variables	Overall Preparedness	Material Preparedness	Behavior Preparedness	Awareness Preparedness
Place attachment	0.34 ***	0.13 ***	0.15 ***	0.08 **
	(0.09)	(0.05)	(0.04)	(0.04)
Self-efficacy	0.53 ***	0.19 ***	0.12 ***	0.22 ***
	(0.08)	(0.04)	(0.03)	(0.03)
Disaster experience	0.23 ***	0.08 ***	0.10 ***	0.05 ***
	(0.04)	(0.02)	(0.02)	(0.02)
Age	−0.02 ***	0.00	−0.01 ***	−0.01 ***
	(0.01)	(0.00)	(0.00)	(0.00)
Child(ren) at home	0.13	0.12	−0.06	0.08
	(0.31)	(0.17)	(0.13)	(0.13)
Gender	0.41 ***	0.14 *	0.12 *	0.14 **
	(0.15)	(0.08)	(0.06)	(0.06)
Ethnicity	0.01	0.68	−0.23	−0.44
	(1.00)	(0.54)	(0.43)	(0.42)
Community (rural/urban)	0.31	0.33 **	0.10	−0.12
	(0.31)	(0.17)	(0.13)	(0.13)
Religion	−0.10	−0.19	0.05	0.03
	(0.30)	(0.16)	(0.13)	(0.13)
Marital status	0.49 **	0.32 ***	0.05	0.11
	(0.19)	(0.10)	(0.08)	(0.08)
Education	0.52 ***	0.13 ***	0.24 ***	0.17 ***
	(0.07)	(0.04)	(0.03)	(0.03)
CPC membership	1.23 ***	0.36 **	0.37 ***	0.51 ***
	(0.26)	(0.14)	(0.11)	(0.11)
Annual household income	0.00 **	0.00	0.00 **	0.00 ***
	(0.00)	(0.00)	(0.00)	(0.00)
Property ownership	−0.26 *	−0.13 *	−0.10	−0.03
	(0.14)	(0.08)	(0.06)	(0.06)
N	1831	1842	1840	1833
R^2	0.19	0.07	0.16	0.16

Note: standard errors in parentheses; *** $p < 0.01$, ** $p < 0.05$, * $p < 0.1$.

One degree's increase of place attachment is positively correlated with a 0.34, 0.13, 0.15, and 0.08 degree of increase in overall disaster preparedness, material preparedness, behavioral preparedness, and awareness preparedness. Thus, Hypothesis 1 is supported, demonstrating that residents with a stronger sense of place attachment prepare more for potential disasters.

Self-efficacy is also associated with a higher degree of overall disaster preparedness ($\beta = 0.53$, $p < 0.01$), material preparedness ($\beta = 0.19$, $p < 0.01$), behavioral preparedness ($\beta = 0.12$, $p < 0.01$) and the awareness preparedness ($\beta = 0.22$, $p < 0.01$). Thus, Hypothesis 2 is supported.

Moreover, the respondents that have disaster experience, with older age, male gender, CPC members, with higher education level, and with higher annual household income tend to have significantly higher levels of disaster preparedness, while the effects of variables such as having at least one child at home, ethnicity, and religious status are not significant. The results also suggest that being married, and living in an urban area tend to indicate a higher degree of material preparedness, but not behavior preparedness and awareness preparedness.

3.3. The Mediation Effect of Self-Efficacy

As shown in Tables 3 and 4, place attachment was positively associated with disaster preparedness and self-efficacy. Meanwhile, self-efficacy was also significantly associated with disaster preparedness, which means the mediating effect of self-efficacy was confirmed between place attachment and all types of preparedness.

Table 4. Test of mediating role of self-efficacy between place attachment and preparedness.

Variables	Overall	Overall	Material	Material	Behavior	Behavior	Awareness	Awareness	Self-Efficacy
Placeattachment	0.42 *** (0.09)		0.16 *** (0.05)		0.17 *** (0.04)		0.11 *** (0.04)		0.15 *** (0.03)
Self-efficacy		0.58 *** (0.08)		0.21 *** (0.04)		0.14 *** (0.03)		0.23 *** (0.03)	
N	1835	1834	1848	1846	1844	1844	1839	1836	1842
R²	0.17	0.18	0.06	0.06	0.16	0.16	0.14	0.16	0.05

Note: Due to the page limitation, the results of the controlled variables were not reported here but are included in Table S1; standard errors in parentheses; *** $p < 0.01$.

We employed the Sobel Goodman test to test the mediating effects of self-efficacy between place attachment and disaster preparedness. We estimated 2000 bootstrap samples in which the independent variable was place attachment, the mediator was self-efficacy, and the dependent variables were emergency preparedness. We also included control variables as covariates in the model. The results indicated that self-efficacy partially mediated the relationship between place attachment and overall disaster preparedness (indirect effect = 0.08; 95% CI: [0.05, 0.11]; direct effect = 0.34, 95% CI: [0.17, 0.51]). Specifically, (1) in the regression of the overall preparedness (dependent variable) and the place attachment (independent variable), the coefficient of place attachment was significant ($\beta = 0.42$, $p < 0.01$). (2) In the regression of self-efficacy (mediator) and the place attachment (independent variable), the coefficient of place attachment was significant ($\beta = 0.15$, $p < 0.01$). (3) In the regression of the overall preparedness (dependent variable) and self-efficacy (independent variable), the coefficient of mediator was significant ($\beta = 0.53$, $p < 0.01$).

Similarly, we tested the mediating roles of self-efficacy between place attachment and the three types of preparedness—the material preparedness, behavioral preparedness and awareness preparedness, respectively. The results demonstrated that self-efficacy partially mediated the relationship between place attachment and material preparedness (indirect effect = 0.03; 95% CI: [0.01, 0.04]; direct effect = 0.13, 95% CI: [0.03, 0.22]), behavior preparedness (indirect effect = 0.02; 95% CI: [0.01, 0.03]; direct effect = 0.15, 95% CI: [0.07, 0.22]), awareness preparedness (indirect effect = 0.03; 95% CI: [0.02, 0.05]; direct effect = 0.08, 95% CI: [0.01, 0.15]). Three step test results of the mediating effects among material preparedness, behavioral preparedness and awareness preparedness were shown in Tables 3 and 4. Accordingly, Hypothesis 3 was supported and the effect for each individual path was illustrated in Figure 3.

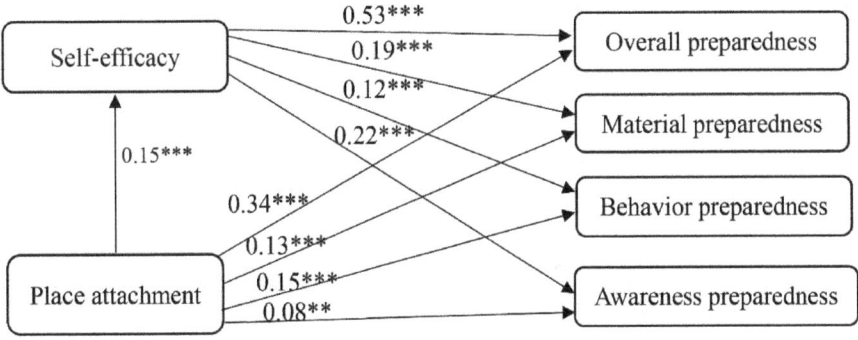

Figure 3. The mediating effect of self-efficacy between place attachment and preparedness. Note: *** $p < 0.01$, ** $p < 0.05$.

4. Discussion

Using representative data from Shandong province, one area that had relatively fewer occurrences of disasters but facing increasing threats of typhoon and flood recently, we analyzed the correlations between place attachment and disaster preparedness, with an effort to examine the mediating role of self-efficacy. This paper has at least the following notable contributions to the current knowledge.

Place attachment is not only positively correlated with the overall degree of disaster preparedness but is also associated with the three dimensions of disaster preparedness, namely the material preparedness, awareness preparedness, and behavioral preparedness, as we assumed in H1. Such a positive correlation is consistent with the prior investigation in India in the context of flood disasters [18], and China in the context of landslide [21], as well as Australia in the context of a wildfire [26], but contradicted the findings from Australia's climate change adaptation [61]. One possible reason is that we did not use the multidimensional measure of place attachment, and the varied dimensions of place attachment, such as place identity, place dependence, neighborhood quality, and detachment [62], may have different or even contradicting effects on preparedness. Emotional attachment may increase people's motivation to protect themselves and the community but make them reluctant to evacuate during emergencies. The familiarity with a community may also diminish people's motivation to take action due to the over-confidence bias [63].

Our analysis also confirms that self-efficacy is positively correlated with disaster preparedness, as most previous studies have demonstrated. Thus, hypothesis II was supported. Moreover, we found that self-efficacy mediated the correlations between place attachment and disaster preparedness, and the path coefficients between place attachment, self-efficacy, overall preparedness, material preparedness, awareness preparedness, and behavior preparedness are statistically significant. Therefore, hypothesis III was also confirmed. Self-efficacy is one of the most critical cognitive variables that link people's understanding of risk and the adoption of actual actions. Although some studies indicated that self-efficacy exerted more influence on planning for preparedness than actual preparedness behaviors [64], this analysis followed the same observations from Mumbai, Taiwan, and Australia [29,34,65]. Besides, we are aware that scholars have proposed several types of efficacies recently, such as the collective efficacy (how community or government can handle the potential disasters effectively) [31,32] or the responsive/outcome efficacy (how effective the actions adopted in disaster risk reduction are in reducing the impact from potential disasters) [28–30]. This paper contributes to our understanding that self-efficacy can directly promote disaster preparedness and play a mediation role between other variables, such as place attachment in this study and the disaster preparedness behaviors.

Additionally, we found that people with a higher level of education and being a CPC member adopted much more preparedness activities in this analysis. This finding highlighted the potential targeted vulnerable group and the household with a lower education level. It could be possible that the under-educated do not know the availability of actions they can adopt to prepare for disasters. Our previous survey about participants' preparedness activities revealed that the majority reason for not preparing for potential disasters was that they were not aware of the existing preparedness activities. In contrast, most of the CPC members are local officials or community leaders in China, and they are usually expected to spearhead the "public desired" actions in the community. Not surprisingly, this group has a more significant potential to access the disaster risk reduction knowledge and resources, and thus, they have a much higher degree of preparedness for disaster.

The findings of this paper have practical implications for disaster risk reduction practice because it investigated the residents from an area with potential typhoons and floods, but they have not had much disaster experience previously. Considering the historical flood threats in this region and the increasing trend of typhoons and floods, this paper highlighted the importance of place attachment and self-efficacy in promoting disaster preparedness activities. Disaster risk reduction outreach programs and advocacies should and could highlight the strong sense of community and also encourage and let the public know their capacity of preparing for disasters, and thus, they can better prepare for potential hazards in the age of uncertainties.

This analysis has at least three limitations. Firstly, the inevitable limitation of the cross-sectional survey in this investigation cannot really solve the causal relations between the variables. Considering the increasing application of experiments, or experiment-embedding in surveys, studies using these new and advanced techniques could be conducted to produce more scientific conclusions in the future. Secondly, this analysis only employed data from a province with relatively fewer occurrences of disasters in China, and thus the overall generalization of this study might be needed. Thirdly, we only included limited dimensions of place attachment and efficacy measures in this analysis; studies including other dimensions of place attachment or types of efficacies such as the collective efficacy and response efficacy [28–32] are needed.

5. Conclusions

This study investigated the associations between place attachment, self-efficacy, and disaster preparedness, and we found that a stronger sense of place attachment predicts higher degrees of all the three types of preparedness, namely the material preparedness, behavioral preparedness, and awareness preparedness. Self-efficacy is also positively correlated with all types of preparedness. Moreover, self-efficacy plays a mediating role between place attachment and disaster preparedness. This study enriched the social cognitive theory in the disaster contexts by investigating the complex relationships between place attachment, self-efficacy and disaster preparedness. These findings highlight the importance of promoting self-efficacy and place attachment in disaster risk reduction advocacies and outreaches. Studies using the experimental method and covering more dimensions of the place attachment and more types of efficacy are needed in future studies.

Supplementary Materials: The following are available online at https://www.mdpi.com/article/10.3390/ijerph18115565/s1, Table S1: Test of mediating role of self-efficacy between place attachment and preparedness with control variables shown.

Author Contributions: Conceptualization, all; data collection and curation, L.L., S.Y.; methodology, Z.W.; validation, Z.W., Z.H.; formal analysis, Z.W.; writing—original draft preparation, Z.W.; writing—review and editing, S.Y., Z.H.; project administration, Z.W., S.Y.; funding acquisition, L.L., S.Y., Z.H. All authors have read and agreed to the published version of the manuscript.

Funding: This research was supported by the National Social Science Foundation of China (20ZD&160), the National Natural Science Foundation of China (72042008), the Fundamental Research Funds for the Central Universities, Shandong University (IFWF2023) and the Graduate Research Fund of PSPA, Shandong University. The funding sources were not involved in the study design, data collection, analysis, interpretation of data, writing of the report, or decision to submit the manuscript for publication.

Institutional Review Board Statement: According to the statement of the Shandong General Social Survey.

Informed Consent Statement: Informed consent was obtained from all subjects involved in the study.

Data Availability Statement: According to the data access policies, the data used to support the findings of this study are available from the Institute of Governance, Shandong University. Reasonable request for SGSS data is available through email: iog@sdu.edu.cn.

Acknowledgments: The authors would like to thank all the participants of the SGSS.

Conflicts of Interest: The authors declare no conflict of interest.

References

1. United Nations Office for Disaster Risk Reduction (UNDRR) Preparedness. Available online: https://www.undrr.org/terminology/preparedness (accessed on 1 February 2021).
2. Kulmala, I.; Salmela, H.; Kalliohaka, T.; Zwęgliński, T.; Smolarkiewicz, M.; Taipale, A.; Kataja, J. A tool for determining sheltering efficiency of mechanically ventilated buildings against outdoor hazardous agents. *Build. Environ.* **2016**, *106*, 245–253. [CrossRef]
3. Kulmala, I.; Zwęgliński, T.; Smolarkiewicz, M.; Salmela, H.; Kalliohaka, T.; Taipale, A.; Kataja, J.; Mäkipää, V. Effect of enhanced supply air filtration in buildings on protecting citizens from environmental radioactive particles. *Build. Simul.* **2020**, *13*, 865–872. [CrossRef]

4. Phillips, B.; Neal, D.M.; Webb, G. *Introduction to Emergency Management*, 2nd ed.; CRC Press: Boca Raton, FL, USA, 2016; ISBN 978-1-4822-4506-6.
5. Haddow, G.D.; Bullock, J.A.; Coppola, D.P. *Introduction to Emergency Management*, 6th ed.; Butterworth-Heinemann: Amsterdam, The Netherlands, 2017; ISBN 978-0-12-803064-6.
6. Wu, G.; Han, Z.; Xu, W.; Gong, Y. Mapping individuals' earthquake preparedness in China. *Nat. Hazards Earth Syst. Sci.* **2018**, *18*, 1315–1325. [CrossRef]
7. Han, Z.; Wang, H.; Du, Q.; Zeng, Y. Natural hazards preparedness in Taiwan: A comparison between households with and without disabled members. *Health Secur.* **2017**, *15*, 575–581. [CrossRef] [PubMed]
8. Lindell, M.K.; Perry, R.W. The protective action decision model: Theoretical modifications and additional evidence. *Risk Anal.* **2011**, *32*, 616–632. [CrossRef] [PubMed]
9. Sadiq, A.-A. Determinants of organizational preparedness for floods: U.S. employees' perceptions. *Risk Hazards Crisis Public Policy* **2017**, *8*, 28–47. [CrossRef]
10. Sadiq, A.-A.; Tharp, K.; Graham, J.D. FEMA versus local governments: Influence and reliance in disaster preparedness. *Nat. Hazards* **2016**, *82*, 123–138. [CrossRef]
11. Sadiq, A.-A.; Tyler, J. Variations in public and private employees' perceptions of organizational preparedness for natural disasters. *Environ. Hazards* **2016**, *15*, 160–177. [CrossRef]
12. Murray, M.; Watson, P.K. Adoption of natural disaster preparedness and risk reduction measures by business organisations in Small island developing states—A Caribbean case study. *Int. J. Disaster Risk Reduct.* **2019**, *39*, 101115. [CrossRef]
13. Multihazard Mitigation Council. *Natural Hazard Mitigation Saves: 2017 Interim Report*; National Institute of Building Science: Washington, DC, USA, 2017.
14. Federal Emergency Management Agency. *A Whole Community Approach to Emergency Management: Principles, Themes, and Pathways for Action*; Federal Emergency Management Agency, US Department of Homeland Security: Washington, DC, USA, 2011.
15. Paton, D. Disaster risk reduction: Psychological perspectives on preparedness. *Aust. J. Psychol.* **2019**, *71*, 327–341. [CrossRef]
16. Paton, D. Disaster preparedness: A social-cognitive perspective. *Disaster Prev. Manag. Int. J.* **2003**, *12*, 210–216. [CrossRef]
17. De Dominicis, S.; Fornara, F.; Cancellieri, U.G.; Twigger-Ross, C.; Bonaiuto, M. We are at risk, and so what? Place attachment, environmental risk perceptions and preventive coping behaviours. *J. Environ. Psychol.* **2015**, *43*, 66–78. [CrossRef]
18. Mishra, S.; Mazumdar, S.; Suar, D. Place attachment and flood preparedness. *J. Environ. Psychol.* **2010**, *30*, 187–197. [CrossRef]
19. Bonaiuto, M.; Alves, S.; De Dominicis, S.; Petruccelli, I. Place attachment and natural hazard risk: Research review and agenda. *J. Environ. Psychol.* **2016**, *48*, 33–53. [CrossRef]
20. Adie, B.A. Place attachment and post-disaster decision-making in a second home context: A conceptual framework. *Curr. Issues Tour.* **2019**, *23*, 1205–1215. [CrossRef]
21. Xu, D.; Peng, L.; Liu, S.; Wang, X. Influences of risk perception and sense of place on landslide disaster preparedness in southwestern China. *Int. J. Disaster Risk Sci.* **2018**, *9*, 167–180. [CrossRef]
22. Bonaiuto, M.; Breakwell, G.M.; Can, I. Identity processes and environmental threat: The effects of nationalism and local identity upon perception of beach pollution. *J. Community Appl. Soc. Psychol.* **1996**, *6*, 157–175. [CrossRef]
23. Gifford, R.; Scannell, L.; Kormos, C.; Smolova, L.; Biel, A.; Boncu, S.; Corral, V.; Güntherf, H.; Hanyu, K.; Hine, D.; et al. Temporal pessimism and spatial optimism in environmental assessments: An 18-nation study. *J. Environ. Psychol.* **2009**, *29*, 1–12. [CrossRef]
24. Swapan, M.S.H.; Sadeque, S. Place attachment in natural hazard-prone areas and decision to relocate: Research review and agenda for developing countries. *Int. J. Disaster Risk Reduct.* **2021**, *52*, 101937. [CrossRef]
25. Ratnam, C.; Drozdzewski, D.D.; Rosalie, D. Can place attachment mediate perceptions of bushfire risk? A case study of the blue mountains, NSW. *Aust. J. Emerg. Manag.* **2016**, *31*, 62–66.
26. Anton, C.E.; Lawrence, C. Does place attachment predict wildfire mitigation and preparedness? A comparison of wildland–urban interface and rural communities. *Environ. Manag.* **2015**, *57*, 148–162. [CrossRef]
27. Bandura, A. Self-efficacy mechanism in human agency. *Am Psychol* **1982**, *32*, 122–147. [CrossRef]
28. Grothmann, T.; Reusswig, F. People at risk of flooding: Why some residents take precautionary action while others do not. *Nat. Hazards* **2006**, *38*, 101–120. [CrossRef]
29. Samaddar, S.; Chatterjee, R.; Misra, B.; Tatano, H. Outcome-expectancy and self-efficacy: Reasons or results of flood preparedness intention? *Int. J. Disaster Risk Reduct.* **2014**, *8*, 91–99. [CrossRef]
30. Van Valkengoed, A.M.; Steg, L. Meta-analyses of factors motivating climate change adaptation behaviour. *Nat. Clim. Chang.* **2019**, *9*, 158–163. [CrossRef]
31. Bandura, A. *Self-Efficacy: The Exercise of Control*; Freeman: New York, NY, USA, 1997; ISBN 978-0716728504.
32. Babcicky, P.; Seebauer, S. Collective efficacy and natural hazards: Differing roles of social cohesion and task-specific efficacy in shaping risk and coping beliefs. *J. Risk Res.* **2019**, *23*, 695–712. [CrossRef]
33. Adams, R.M.; Eisenman, D.P.; Glik, D. Community advantage and individual self-efficacy promote disaster preparedness: A multilevel model among persons with disabilities. *Int. J. Environ. Res. Public Health* **2019**, *16*, 2779. [CrossRef]
34. Tang, J.-S.; Feng, J.-Y. Residents' disaster preparedness after the meinong taiwan earthquake: A test of protection motivation theory. *Int. J. Environ. Res. Public Health* **2018**, *15*, 1434. [CrossRef] [PubMed]
35. Yu, J.; Sim, T.; Qi, W.; Zhu, Z. Communication with local officials, self-efficacy, and individual disaster preparedness: A case study of rural northwestern China. *Sustainability* **2020**, *12*, 5354. [CrossRef]

36. Bubeck, P.; Botzen, W.J.W.; Laudan, J.; Aerts, J.C.; Thieken, A.H. Insights into flood-coping appraisals of protection motivation theory: Empirical evidence from germany and france. *Risk Anal.* **2017**, *38*, 1239–1257. [CrossRef]
37. Richert, C.; Erdlenbruch, K.; Figuières, C. The determinants of households' flood mitigation decisions in France—On the possibility of feedback effects from past investments. *Ecol. Econ.* **2017**, *131*, 342–352. [CrossRef]
38. Botzen, W.J.W.; Kunreuther, H.; Czajkowski, J.; De Moel, H. Adoption of individual flood damage mitigation measures in New York City: An extension of protection motivation theory. *Risk Anal.* **2019**, *39*, 2143–2159. [CrossRef] [PubMed]
39. Seebauer, S.; Babcicky, P. The sources of belief in personal capability: Antecedents of self-efficacy in private adaptation to flood risk. *Risk Anal.* **2020**, *40*, 1967–1982. [CrossRef] [PubMed]
40. Rostami-Moez, M.; Rabiee-Yeganeh, M.; Shokouhi, M.; Dosti-Irani, A.; Rezapur-Shahkolai, F. Earthquake preparedness of households and its predictors based on health belief model. *BMC Public Health* **2020**, *20*, 646–648. [CrossRef] [PubMed]
41. Hallak, R.; Assaker, G.; Lee, C. Tourism entrepreneurship performance: The effects of place identity, self-efficacy, and gender. *J. Travel Res.* **2013**, *54*, 36–51. [CrossRef]
42. Twigger-Ross, C.L.; Uzzell, D. Place and identity processes. *J. Environ. Psychol.* **1996**, *16*, 205–220. [CrossRef]
43. Anton, C.E.; Lawrence, C. Home is where the heart is: The effect of place of residence on place attachment and community participation. *J. Environ. Psychol.* **2014**, *40*, 451–461. [CrossRef]
44. Knez, I. Attachment and identity as related to a place and its perceived climate. *J. Environ. Psychol.* **2005**, *25*, 207–218. [CrossRef]
45. Wang, B.; Song, L.; Sun, N. Study on natural disasters and their impact since ming and qing dynasties—A case study of shandong province (1368–1949). *J. Qingdao Agric. Univ. Soc. Sci.* **2012**, *24*, 74–79. (In Chinese)
46. Wang, J.; Liu, H.; Cao, J.; Qiu, C. Analysis on the main disaster characteristics in Shandong province from 1984 to 2013. *Meteorol. J. Inn. Mong.* **2015**, *5*, 53–56. (In Chinese)
47. Lu, X.; Yu, H.; Ying, M.; Zhao, B.; Zhang, S.; Lin, L.; Bai, L.; Wan, R. Western north pacific tropical cyclone database created by the china meteorological administration. *Adv. Atmos. Sci.* **2021**, *38*, 690–699. [CrossRef]
48. Ying, M.; Zhang, W.; Yu, H.; Lu, X.; Feng, J.; Fan, Y.; Zhu, Y.; Chen, D. An overview of the china meteorological administration tropical cyclone database. *J. Atmos. Ocean. Technol.* **2014**, *31*, 287–301. [CrossRef]
49. China Meteorological Administration Tropical Cyclone Data Center. Available online: http://tcdata.typhoon.org.cn/ (accessed on 30 March 2021).
50. Sha, J. The Typhoon Caused a Direct Economic Loss of 9.2 Billion Yuan to More than 1.47 Million People in Weifang, Shandong. Available online: http://www.chinanews.com/gn/2018/08-23/8608820.shtml (accessed on 1 February 2021).
51. Xie, C. Typhoon Lekima Batters Shandong Province. Available online: https://www.chinadaily.com.cn/a/201908/12/WS5d5105fba310cf3e355653a8.html (accessed on 1 February 2021).
52. Hong, Y.; Kim, J.-S.; Xiong, L. Media exposure and individuals' emergency preparedness behaviors for coping with natural and human-made disasters. *J. Environ. Psychol.* **2019**, *63*, 82–91. [CrossRef]
53. Hoffmann, R.; Muttarak, R. Learn from the Past, prepare for the future: Impacts of education and experience on disaster preparedness in the Philippines and Thailand. *World Dev.* **2017**, *96*, 32–51. [CrossRef]
54. Tam, G.; Huang, Z.; Chan, E.Y.Y. Household preparedness and preferred communication channels in public health emergencies: A cross-sectional survey of residents in an asian developed urban city. *Int. J. Environ. Res. Public Health* **2018**, *15*, 1598. [CrossRef]
55. Sattler, D.N.; Kaiser, C.F.; Hittner, J.B. Disaster preparedness: Relationships among prior experience, personal characteristics, and distress[1]. *J. Appl. Soc. Psychol.* **2000**, *30*, 1396–1420. [CrossRef]
56. Josephson, A.; Schrank, H.; Marshall, M. Assessing preparedness of small businesses for hurricane disasters: Analysis of pre-disaster owner, business and location characteristics. *Int. J. Disaster Risk Reduct.* **2017**, *23*, 25–35. [CrossRef]
57. Han, Z.; Lu, X.; Hörhager, E.I.; Yan, J. The effects of trust in government on earthquake survivors' risk perception and preparedness in China. *Nat. Hazards* **2017**, *86*, 437–452. [CrossRef]
58. Han, Z.; Wang, L.; Cui, K. Trust in Stakeholders and Social Support: Risk Perception and Preparedness by the Wenchuan Earthquake Survivors. *Environ. Hazards* **2021**, *20*, 132–145. [CrossRef]
59. MacKinnon, D.P.; Lockwood, C.M.; Hoffman, J.M.; West, S.G.; Sheets, V. A comparison of methods to test mediation and other intervening variable effects. *Psychol. Methods* **2002**, *7*, 83–104. [CrossRef]
60. Wen, Z.; Chang, L.; Hau, K.-T.; Liu, H. Testing and application of the mediating effects. *Acta Psychol. Sin.* **2004**, *36*, 614–620. (In Chinese)
61. Marshall, N.A.; Dowd, A.-M.; Fleming, A.; Gambley, C.; Howden, M.; Jakku, S.; Larsen, C.; Marshall, P.A.; Moon, K.; Park, S.; et al. Transformational capacity in Australian peanut farmers for better climate adaptation. *Agron. Sustain. Dev.* **2014**, *34*, 583–591. [CrossRef]
62. Greer, A.; Binder, S.B.; Thiel, A.; Jamali, M.; Nejat, A. Place attachment in disaster studies: Measurement and the case of the 2013 moore tornado. *Popul. Environ.* **2020**, *41*, 306–329. [CrossRef]
63. Levy, J.S. An introduction to prospect theory. *Political Psychol.* **1992**, *13*, 171–186.
64. Wirtz, P.W.; Rohrbeck, C.A. The dynamic role of perceived threat and self-efficacy in motivating terrorism preparedness behaviors. *Int. J. Disaster Risk Reduct.* **2018**, *27*, 366–372. [CrossRef]
65. Kanakis, K. Preparing for disaster: Preparedness in a flood and cyclone prone community. *Aust. J. Emerg. Manag.* **2016**, *31*, 7.

Article

Will Anti-Epidemic Campus Signals Affect College Students' Preparedness in the Post-COVID-19 Era?

Teng Zhao [1], Yuchen Zhang [2], Chao Wu [3] and Qiang Su [1,*]

1. Zhejiang Academy of Higher Education, Hangzhou Dianzi University, Hangzhou 310018, China; zhaoteng@hdu.edu.cn
2. Chinese Academy of Science and Education Evaluation, Hangzhou Dianzi University, Hangzhou 310018, China; zyc@hdu.edu.cn
3. Propaganda Department, Hangzhou Dianzi University, Hangzhou 310018, China; we926@hdu.edu.cn
* Correspondence: xsdsq@163.com

Abstract: The COVID-19 pandemic has been a tremendous global threat and challenge for human beings, and individuals need to be prepared for the next wave of the outbreak, especially in the educational setting. Limited research has focused on individual knowledge, awareness, and preparedness of COVID-19 in postsecondary institutions in the post-COVID-19 era so far. This study aimed to explore whether students' perceived anti-epidemic campus signals had effects on their awareness of and preparedness for COVID-19. Leveraging the data collected from full-time college students in a province located in East China and building a structural regression model, we found that students' perceived anti-epidemic campus signals were significantly associated with their awareness of and preparedness for COVID-19. With one perceived signal decrease, there were 0.099 unit and 0.051 unit decreases in students' awareness and preparedness, respectively. In addition, we indeed found that female students had a higher awareness and better preparedness than their male peers. These findings provided important implications for postsecondary administrators and policymakers, as well as future research.

Keywords: COVID-19; campus signal; disaster preparedness; disaster awareness; structural regression model

1. Introduction

The COVID-19 pandemic has been a tremendous global threat and challenge for human beings. According to the Coronavirus Resource Center at Johns Hopkins University, to date, more than 172 million cases and 3.7 million deaths have been reported across the world [1]. The strong infectiousness requires people to keep social distance, which has challenged the education system [2]. All levels of educational institutions, such as secondary schools and postsecondary institutions, were shut down temporarily and shifted to online courses during the peak of the pandemic. With the massive efforts endowed by governments and the people, COVID-19 in China has been effectively controlled, and the education system has also returned to normal operation. However, since the pandemic is still far from over, necessary preparations to prevent the infection and spread of the virus are needed.

Previous research has found that physical school environments could significantly affect student behavior [3,4]. For example, Johnson found that a positive school environment can increase perceived fairness and, thus, reduce school violence [5]. As such, college students' perception of the anti-epidemic tension released by universities may influence their awareness of the pandemic. This is also partially consistent with Tkachuck et al.'s view that students' perceived university preparedness was positively associated with disaster concern [6].

In China, as the majority of college students live on campus, they are likely to observe and experience campus changes, such as campus policy changes (e.g., social distance policy and health code policy) and physical environment changes (e.g., separators on the dining tables and banners in campus cafeterias). These are signals that deliver important campus messages to students to inform them that something may happen. Especially at this particular time, universities and colleges require students to stay on campus more, which itself could be regarded as a signal that students still need to be aware of the pandemic.

The reality is, as China quickly enters the post-COVID-19 era, though the overall anti-epidemic work is effective, there are still sporadic and recurrent outbreaks in some places, which periodically alert the whole nation. Campus anti-epidemic policies and/or measures are appropriately adjusted in terms of the actual national situation of the epidemic. When the pandemic is well controlled, in general, campuses have loose anti-epidemic actions; inversely, if the pandemic has signs of resurgence, campuses will immediately be put on alert and take anti-epidemic actions. In this study, we refer to these kinds of anti-epidemic actions as anti-epidemic campus signals that deliver messages to students to inform them of the severity of the pandemic. These campus signals are likely to influence students' preparation awareness of COVID-19. For instance, when a campus has strict anti-epidemic policies, it may increase students' preparation awareness. On the contrary, a campus with undemanding anti-epidemic policies may decrease it.

This study seeks to better understand whether anti-epidemic campus signals affect college students' preparedness of COVID-19. This is crucial for research literature, as well as having practical implications. Past studies only theoretically suggest how educational institutions prevent COVID-19 [2] and suggest recommendations for medical students' COVID-19 preparedness [7,8]. To our knowledge, there is no existing literature that analyzes the relationship between anti-epidemic campus signals and students' COVID-19 preparedness. As a consequence, there is insufficient empirical evidence to inform postsecondary administrators and policy makers of whether anti-epidemic campus signals contribute to increasing students' COVID-19 preparedness, even in a relatively safe situation. Leveraging the data collected from the survey of College Students' Epidemic Preparedness in Post-COVID-19 Era (CSEPPCE), we examine the relationship between campus signals and college students' preparedness with structural equation models.

2. Literature Review

2.1. Research on Knowledge, Awareness, and Preparedness in Disaster Management

Researchers have documented how preparedness is important for disaster management [9]. Experiences from past disasters affirm that pre-disaster preparedness can effectively reduce the loss brought by disasters and shorten milling processes. For example, the 1994 Northridge quake in Southern California that quickly reached a stable condition largely relied on residents' being well-informed about earthquake preparedness [10]. In fact, better grasping the knowledge of disasters, such as what the disaster is and what the mechanism of the disaster is, and having a stronger awareness of disasters, such as the perception of risk, contribute to better preparedness.

The existing research has found that disaster knowledge and awareness of disasters are strongly associated with disaster preparedness [11–14]. Yu et al. applied a moderated mediation model using data collected from 1080 villagers in Shanxi province and found that the positive relationship between villagers' disaster preparedness and communication with local officials was mediated by their disaster knowledge [11]. Using residents' data from the hazard-threatened areas located in the Three Gorges Reservoir area and conducting regression models, Xu et al. found that residents with higher risk perception were more likely to adopt preparedness for a sudden landslide [15].

Specifically, in the circumstance of our study, COVID-19, we hypothesized the following:

Hypothesis 1. *Students who have better knowledge of COVID-19 will be better prepared.*

Hypothesis 2. *Students with higher awareness of COVID-19 will be better prepared.*

Comprehensively understanding disaster risks, one of the categories of disaster knowledge [16], ought to increase individuals' awareness. The relationship between disaster knowledge and awareness has also been investigated in the prior literature. Interviewing 50 secondary students, Pinar suggested that disaster education that contributes to students' knowledge of the disaster needs to be carried out by different stakeholders in order to raise their awareness [17]. Furthermore, some literature [18–20] has focused on disaster education programs and/or training, which can increase students' knowledge of disasters, to examine whether disaster knowledge is associated with awareness. For instance, Ozkazanc and Yuksel found that students who received disaster training have a significantly higher awareness of disasters [20].

Specifically, in the circumstance of our study, COVID-19, we hypothesized the following:

Hypothesis 3. *Students who have a better knowledge of COVID-19 will have a higher awareness of COVID-19.*

In addition, disaster knowledge, awareness, and preparedness may also vary among different groups of the population. Eisenman et al. illustrated that Latinos were at a relatively lower level of disaster knowledge and preparedness [21]. Elliott and Pais found that Blacks were more likely to be evacuated after the storm, rather than before the storm, compared to similar Whites [22], indicating that Blacks may have a lower risk perception or awareness. According to these findings, it seems that socially underrepresented groups have a lower disaster knowledge, awareness, and preparedness. Kohn et al. reviewed 36 studies and found that different groups of the population had different disaster preparedness [12]. Cvetković et al. found that men perceived greater preparedness at both the individual and household level after the flooding [23].

Specifically, in the circumstance of our study, COVID-19, we hypothesized the following:

Hypothesis 4. *Male students have a higher awareness of COVID-19 and are more likely to be better prepared than their female peers.*

Hypothesis 5. *Han students, as the socially dominant group in China, have a higher awareness of COVID-19 and are more likely to be better prepared than their peers of other ethnicities.*

Guided by the above literature, our study examines whether the relationships between knowledge and preparedness, between awareness and preparedness, and between knowledge and awareness also apply to college students at this particular moment in the post-COVID-19 era. Additionally, we investigated whether there are variations between different gender groups and ethnicity groups. This study is extremely important because gatherings in postsecondary institutions may accelerate the spread of COVID-19, and better understanding the factors that influence students' preparedness for COVID-19 is crucial. Considering COVID-19 is a type of disaster, we expected a similar pattern in these relationships compared to other types of disaster, such as landslides and earthquakes.

2.2. Research on Signals, Awareness, and Preparedness in Disaster Management

Studies exploring the effect of signals on individuals' awareness and preparedness are relatively scarce. The majority of this research has focused on warning signals and has aimed to analyze the influence of such signals on individuals' awareness and preparedness [24–26]. These warning signals delivered to the public through media contribute to people's perception of disaster risks and preparedness [26]. Currently, generally, if a disaster can be detected, warning signals will be provided by authorities before the disaster. However, unlike other disasters, COVID-19 outbreaks cannot be precisely predicted. A better approach is to increase risk perception and regular anti-epidemic preparedness [27]. In an extreme scenario, if authorities enforce the public to adopt anti-epidemic measures, such as wearing masks, the public may increase in COVID-19 awareness and make adequate preparations.

From a business management perspective, Bazerman and Hoffman elaborated that individuals can be affected by their perceptions of the environment of the organizations to which they belong [28]. Similarly, in an education setting, college students in postsecondary education may perceive the anti-epidemic campus context, and their awareness and preparedness of COVID-19 may be influenced. Little was known as to whether anti-epidemic measures taken by campuses would influence students' awareness and preparedness for the next potential wave of the outbreak. The anti-epidemic measures required by campuses have changed in terms of COVID-19, and this provides a unique opportunity to investigate whether the anti-epidemic campus signals influence students' awareness and preparedness of COVID-19. Thus, we hypothesized the following:

Hypothesis 6. *A perceived reduction in anti-epidemic campus signals will decrease their awareness of COVID-19.*

Hypothesis 7. *A perceived reduction in anti-epidemic campus signals will weaken their preparedness.*

Filling the gaps in the literature, the purpose of our study is to evaluate the impact of anti-epidemic campus signals on students' preparedness of COVID-19, and to examine the relationships among knowledge, awareness, and preparedness in the COVID-19 pandemic in an educational setting. In other words, we seek to test the aforementioned hypotheses.

3. Methods

3.1. Data Sources and Participants

Guided by Ikhlaq et al. [29] and Ahmed et al. [30], we carefully designed the survey, entitled *College Students' Epidemic Preparedness in Post-COVID-19 Era*, which was randomly distributed to full-time college students in a province located on the east coast of China. The questionnaires mainly focused on students' knowledge, awareness, and preparedness of COVID-19, as well as the anti-epidemic campus signals they perceived. Several items were designed to measure students' knowledge, awareness, and preparedness to more precisely represent these complex and multifaceted variables (see details in Table 1).

The survey was distributed to 1600 full-time college students from 13 postsecondary institutions on May 2021 via WJX.CN, a platform that enables individuals to design surveys and then share survey links to intended participants. We recruited faculties from these postsecondary institutions to help us to share the survey link. The final response rate was 91.88%, yielding a sample of 1470. There were only a few responses to certain survey items missing, so we applied a listwise deletion technique to deal with such missingness, yielding a final analytic sample of 1464. Among them, 690 (47.13%) students were female, and 774 (52.87%) were male. In terms of ethnicity, 1372 (93.72%) were Han, and 92 (6.28%) were of other ethnicities.

3.2. Measures

3.2.1. Endogenous Variables

In our model, one endogenous variable, students' preparedness for COVID-19 in the current period, was measured by three survey items; that is, "will you wear a surgical mask when going outside?", "will you use hand sanitizer?", and "will you keep social distance when you are in public?". They were all constructed on a five-point Likert scale with 1 = "Never" and 5 = "Always". The mean of each item was 2.21, 2.24, and 2.23, respectively, which ranged between "Sometimes" and "Neutral" (see Table 2).

Another was students' awareness of COVID-19, which was measured by seven items on a five-point Likert scale in the survey. However, after the initial check of correlations among these items, four items with low correlations were dropped from the analysis. The remaining three items were "how often will you talk about COVID-19 with your classmates", "how often will you talk about COVID-19 with your friends", and "how often will you talk about COVID-19 with your family", where means = 2.37, 2.26, and 2.29, respectively.

Table 1. Description of variables.

Variable	Variable Description	Variable Type
Endogenous variable		
Awareness		
	Talk about COVID-19 with your classmates and/or roommates	Categorical Variable
	Talk about COVID-19 with your friends	Categorical Variable
	Talk about COVID-19 with your family	Categorical Variable
	Items were measured by a 5-point Likert scales with 5 = Always, 1 = Never	
Preparedness		
	Wear surgical mask when going to class, attending school activities, etc.	Categorical Variable
	The frequency of using hand sanitizer	Categorical Variable
	Keep social distance when in public places	Categorical Variable
	Items were measured by a 5-point Likert scales with 5 = Always, 1 = Never	
Exogenous variable		
Perceived campus signals	Students' perceived changes in anti-epidemic campus signals at the peak of the pandemic and post-COVID-19 era	Continuous Variable
Knowledge		
	You know about the symptoms of COVID-19	Categorical Variable
	You know about how COVID-19 is spread	Categorical Variable
	You know about the anti-epidemic measures of COVID-19	Categorical Variable
	You know about the differences between COVID-19 and other pandemics	Categorical Variable
	Items were measured by a 5-point Likert scales with 5 = extremely familiar, 1 = Not at all familiar	
Control variable		
Male	Whether a student is male or not (1 = Yes, 0 = No)	Dichotomous Variable
Han	Whether a student's ethnicity is Han or not (1 = Yes, 0 = No)	Dichotomous Variable

3.2.2. Exogenous Variables

The perceived change of anti-epidemic campus signals was measured by students' perceived anti-epidemic campus signals in the peak of the outbreak minus students' perceived anti-epidemic campus signals in the current stage. When designing the survey, we carefully checked with recruited faculties on the anti-epidemic campus signals that their own institutions had and selected representative signals that closely related to students' daily life to ensure that surveyed students would easily recognize these signals. These included separators on the dining table, anti-epidemic banners, hand sanitizer in public areas, strict leaving school management, social distancing during classes, the integration of online and face-to-face classes, social distancing in public areas, and school health codes. Different campuses have different anti-epidemic measures, so students from different campuses may experience different anti-epidemic signals. Even on the same campus, the anti-epidemic tension perceived by students may be different. Thus, it is reasonable to use students' perceived change of anti-epidemic campus signals to represent the perceived anti-epidemic tension on campus. Table 2 shows that the mean of students' perceived change of anti-epidemic campus signals was 2.76, indicating that students did feel that campus anti-epidemic measures were suspended in the post-COVID-19 area when compared to the peak of the outbreak.

Students' knowledge of COVID-19, as another exogenous variable, comprised four survey items, also on a five-point Likert scale. We asked: "whether you know about the symptoms of COVID-19", "whether you know how COVID-19 is spread", "whether you know the anti-epidemic measures of COVID-19", and "whether you know the differences between COVID-19 and other pandemics such as SARS", with 1 = "Not at all familiar" and 5 = "Extremely familiar". The mean of each item was 2.93, 3.07, 3.16, and 2.66, respectively.

Table 2. Descriptive statistics of variables.

Variables	Analytic Sample (n = 1464)			
	Mean	SD	Min	Max
Campus Signals				
Perceived campus signals	2.76	1.99	−2	7
Demographic Characteristics				
Male	0.53	0.50	0	1
Female	0.47	0.50	0	1
Han	0.94	0.24	0	1
Others	0.06	0.24	0	1
Knowledge of COVID-19				
Know about COVID-19	2.93	0.92	1	5
Know how COVID-19 is spread	3.07	0.93	1	5
Know anti-epidemic measures	3.16	0.91	1	5
Know differences	2.66	1.00	1	5
Awareness of COVID-19				
Talk about COVID-19 with classmates	2.37	0.80	1	5
Talk about COVID-19 with friends	2.26	0.75	1	5
Talk about COVID-19 with family	2.29	0.77	1	5
Preparedness of COVID-19				
Surgical mask	2.21	0.92	1	5
Hand sanitizer	2.24	0.95	1	5
Social distance	2.23	0.87	1	5

3.3. Analytic Plan

First, descriptive statistics were provided as in Table 2 to display the basic information about variables, using Stata 16. Second, correlations between each variable were analyzed to help us select appropriate survey items to measure our latent variables (i.e., knowledge, awareness, and preparedness).

Third, we adopted a two-step approach, suggested by Anderson and Gerbing [31], to assess the fitness of our full structural regression model using Mplus 8 [32]. In the first step, the measurement model was evaluated to assess its adequacy. Applying a diagonally weighted least squares estimator with mean and variance adjusted (WLSMV) based on the polychoric correlation matrix [33], we conducted step-wise measurement model comparisons until the final measurement model was adequate, judging by model fit indices such as the root mean square error of approximation (RMSEA), the standardized root means square residual (SRMR), the comparative fit index (CFI), and the Tucker–Lewis fit index (TLI). In addition to these indices, we also performed a chi-square (χ^2) different test to compare which model was a better fit and then proceeded to the second step. In the second step, we evaluated the adequacy of structural components by comparing the fitness of the structural model to the fitness of the final measurement model until it was adequate. The major relationships that were tested were: (1) the perceived change in campus signals and awareness, (2) the perceived change in campus signals and preparedness, (3) knowledge and preparedness, (4) knowledge and awareness, and (5) awareness and preparedness.

Fourth, in order to understand whether students' demographic characteristics, such as gender and ethnicity, would also influence students' preparedness of COVID-19, we further set gender and ethnicity as control variables in the final structural regression model.

4. Results

4.1. Correlation Results

Table 3 showed the correlations among survey items. Among them, Items 2–5 demonstrated high correlations with a range from 0.69 to 0.87. The correlations among Items 6–8 were from 0.81 to 0.87, and Items 9–10 were from 0.56 to 0.61. These relatively high polychoric correlations provided evidence for us to use these survey items to measure our latent factors: knowledge, awareness, and preparedness, respectively.

Table 3. Correlations between variables for analysis of a structural regression model.

Variables	1	2	3	4	5	6	7	8	9	10	11
Campus Signals											
1. Perceived campus signals	1.00										
Knowledge of COVID-19											
2. Know about COVID-19	−0.01	1.00									
3. Know how COVID-19 is spread	0.01	0.84	1.00								
4. Know anti-epidemic measures	0.00	0.79	0.87	1.00							
5. Know differences	−0.07	0.73	0.73	0.69	1.00						
Awareness of COVID-19											
6. Talk about COVID-19 with classmates	−0.16	0.25	0.20	0.22	0.20	1.00					
7. Talk about COVID-19 with friends	−0.22	0.22	0.16	0.19	0.21	0.87	1.00				
8. Talk about COVID-19 with family	−0.20	0.24	0.18	0.21	0.20	0.81	0.83	1.00			
Preparedness of COVID-19											
9. Surgical mask	−0.18	0.22	0.19	0.18	0.31	0.34	0.36	0.34	1.00		
10. Hand sanitizer	−0.14	0.26	0.24	0.28	0.35	0.32	0.37	0.37	0.58	1.00	
11. Social distance	−0.19	0.27	0.23	0.25	0.36	0.30	0.38	0.36	0.56	0.61	1.00

NOTE: The correlations among Variables 2–11 are polychoric correlations due to the nature of ordinal variables.

4.2. Two-Step Approach Results

4.2.1. Measurement Model Results

Following Anderson and Gerbing's two-step approach [31], we then tested the measurement model associated with our full structural model, denoted as the initial model in Table 4. According to the cutoff values of the model fit indices recommended by Hu and Bentler [34], the initial model demonstrated a reasonable fit with χ^2 (42) = 444.86, CFI = 0.990, TLI = 0.988, RMSEA = 0.081, and SRMR = 0.051. The model modification indices provided by Mplus software suggested correlations between errors of certain survey items. Upon the consideration of the real meaning of survey items, knowing how COVID-19 is spread helps to know anti-epidemic measures, we applied a step-wise measurement model comparison procedure by adding the correlated error between Items 3 and 4 into our first adjusted measurement model, yielding a better model fit with χ^2 (41) = 403.14, CFI = 0.991, TLI = 0.989, RMSEA = 0.078, and SRMR = 0.050. Considering that students who are well informed about COVID-19 may know the differences between COVID-19 and other pandemics, we then added the correlated error between Items 2 and 5 into the first adjusted measurement model, yielding an even better model fit with χ^2 (40) = 374.37, CFI = 0.992, TLI = 0.989, RMSEA = 0.076, and SRMR = 0.048.

To further affirm which model was statistically better, we conducted a chi-square difference test between the initial model and the adjusted models. We found that in the third model with the correlated errors of Items 3 and 4 and Items 2 and 5, compared to the initial model, the chi-square difference was $\Delta\chi^2 = 70.49$, $p < 0.01$, indicating that the third model outperforms the initial model.

Table 4. A step-wise measurement model comparison procedure and an evaluation of the structural part of the SR model.

	Model	CFI	TLI	RMSEA	SRMR	χ^2	df	$\Delta\chi^2$	Δdf
	Measurement models								
1.	Initial model	0.990	0.988	0.081	0.051	444.86	42		
2.	Spreading mechanisms with anti-epidemic measures	0.991	0.989	0.078	0.050	403.14	41	41.72 *	1
3.	COVID-19 with Differences	0.992	0.989	0.076	0.048	374.37	40	70.49 *	2
	Structural part of the model								
4.	Full structural model	0.998	0.997	0.038	0.022	119.67	38	254.7 *	2

NOTE: * $p < 0.01$. CFI = comparative fit index; TLI = non-normed fit index; RMSEA = root mean square error of approximation; SRMR = standardized root means square residual.

4.2.2. Structural Model Results

After we were satisfied with our adjusted measurement model, we evaluated the structural part of the full structural regression model. The full structural model yielded a good model fit with χ^2 (38) = 119.67, CFI = 0.998, TLI = 0.997, RMSEA = 0.038, and SRMR = 0.022. To assess the fit of the structural part of the model, we also conducted a chi-square difference test and obtained $\Delta\chi^2 = 254.7$, $p < 0.01$ (See Table 4), indicating that the structural part of the model was adequate.

We acquired our final full structural regression model, as presented in Figure 1. Figure 1 shows that the standardized factor loadings for students' knowledge of COVID-19 ranged from 0.819 to 1.013. Jöreskog pointed out that standardized factor loadings can exceed 1.00 and do not necessarily imply a wrong result [35]. The ranges of standardized factor loadings were from 0.880 to 0.947 and from 0.722 to 0.792, respectively, for students' awareness of COVID-19 and students' preparedness for COVID-19. These relatively high factor loadings suggested that three latent factors were well explained by the respective survey items. For example, for the item "know how COVID-19 is spread", the corresponding r square value was 0.671, meaning that 67.1% of the variance in "know how COVID-19 is spread" was explained by students' knowledge of COVID-19.

Looking at the paths in the structural regression model, we found that one unit increasing in students' knowledge of COVID-19 was associated with a 0.210 unit increase in students' preparedness for COVID-19. Thus, Hypothesis 1 was accepted. We also found that students' awareness of COVID-19 was positively and significantly associated with their preparedness ($\beta = 0.310$, $p < 0.001$), which supported Hypothesis 2. Furthermore, the relationship between students' knowledge and preparedness was also positively statistically significant ($\beta = 0.232$, $p < 0.001$); therefore, Hypothesis 3 was accepted.

Focusing on our primary interest of variables, students' perceived anti-epidemic campus signals, we found that when students perceived that an anti-epidemic campus signal was decreasing, there was a 0.099 decrease in their awareness of COVID-19, which proves Hypothesis 6. Not surprisingly, a signal perceived as decreasing by students was associated with a 0.051 decrease in their preparedness. Thus, Hypothesis 7 was supported.

4.3. Structural Regression Model with Controls

As shown in Table 5, when controlling gender and ethnicity in the structural regression model, the model fit indices indicated a good fit, with χ^2 (51) = 205.33, CFI = 0.997, TLI = 0.995, RMSEA = 0.045, and SRMR = 0.021. Compared with the model without gender and ethnicity controls (Model 1), the path coefficients of the model with controls (Model 2) remained statistically significant and in the same directions. Focusing on gender, male students had a lower awareness ($\beta = -0.163$, $p < 0.01$) and preparedness ($\beta = -0.113$, $p < 0.01$) of COVID-19 than their female peers. No evidence was found that students' ethnicities would contribute to their awareness and preparedness. Therefore, both Hypotheses 4 and 5 were rejected.

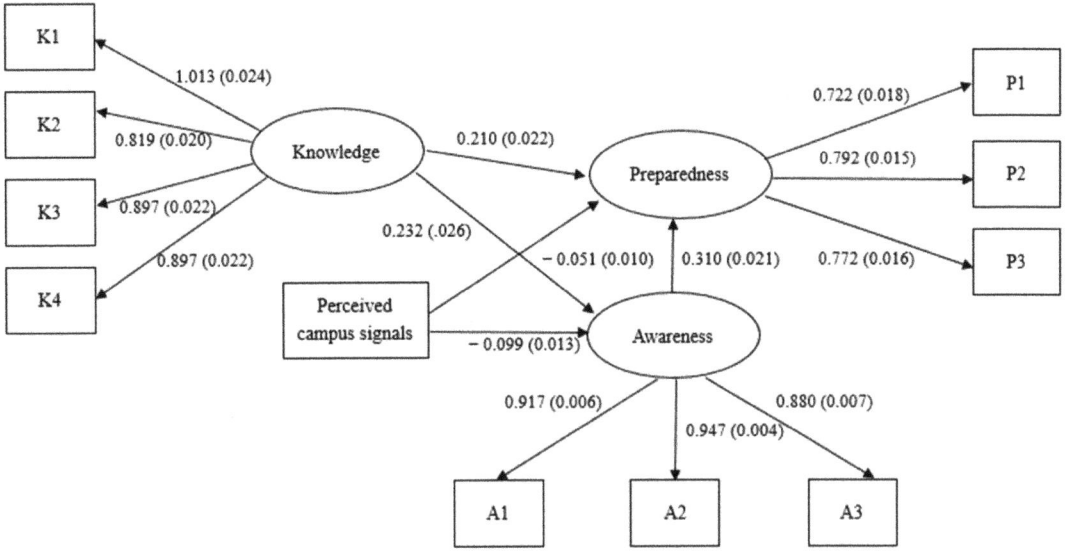

Figure 1. Final full structural regression model of students' perceived anti-epidemic campus signals on their COVID-19 preparedness. Note: The factor loadings were reported by using standardized results, while the path coefficients were reported by using unstandardized results for an easier interpretation; standard errors are in parentheses.

Table 5. Full structural regression model of students' perceived anti-epidemic campus signals on their COVID-19 preparedness with control variables.

Paths		Model 1		Model 2	
		β	SE	β	SE
	Paths to Preparedness				
	1. Knowledge → Preparedness	0.210 ***	0.022	0.210 ***	0.022
	2. Perceived signals → Preparedness	−0.051 ***	0.010	−0.048 ***	0.010
	3. Awareness → Preparedness	0.310 ***	0.021	0.312 ***	0.022
	Paths to Awareness				
	4. Knowledge → Awareness	0.232 ***	0.026	0.229 ***	0.026
	5. Perceived signals → Awareness	−0.099 ***	0.013	−0.093 ***	0.012
	Controls				
	6. Male → Preparedness			−0.113 **	0.038
	7. Male → Awareness			−0.163 **	0.050
	8. Han → Preparedness			0.048	0.070
	9. Han → Awareness			0.165	0.097
	Model fit indices				
	CFI	0.998		0.997	
	TLI	0.997		0.995	
	RMSEA	0.038		0.045	
	SRMR	0.022		0.021	

NOTE: ** $p < 0.01$, *** $p < 0.001$. CFI = comparative fit index; TLI = non-normed fit index; RMSEA = root mean square error of approximation; SRMR = standardized root means square residual.

5. Discussions

Building upon the previous literature, this study utilized the survey data to investigate how anti-epidemic campus signals affect students' preparedness for the COVID-19 pandemic. Signals have been found to make individuals aware of risks before and/or after disasters [26,36]. In an educational setting, we indeed found that these signals could increase students' awareness and contribute to a better preparedness for COVID-19. In addition to this, we also found that students who had more knowledge of COVID-19 were more likely to have a higher awareness and declare better preparedness. In addition, we found that students with a higher awareness were more likely to have better preparedness. Notably, gender was observed to have an influence on students' awareness and preparedness, while ethnicity was not.

Cahapay believed that preparedness for COVID-19 is a priority of education in the post-COVID-19 era [37]. Exploring the factors that influence students' preparedness of COVID-19 is crucial. Our findings showed that students' knowledge and awareness all statistically significantly predict their preparedness. These findings are consistent with Nindrea et al. [38], showing that breast cancer patients' COVID-19 knowledge and awareness were significantly associated with their preparedness. With respect to anti-epidemic campus signals, to our knowledge, no study has focused on this. However, Peng et al. demonstrated that the national anti-epidemic measures effectively help to reduce the reported number of confirmed cases [39], which helps to show that individuals are prepared for COVID-19, partially due to the perceived severities of the pandemic, which is a result of the nation's response to the pandemic. As such, if postsecondary institutions implement strict anti-epidemic measures on campuses, students may have a stronger awareness of COVID-19 and make better preparations. This is supported by our structural regression model.

With respect to the demographic characteristics' influence, past studies have found that gender and race/ethnicity have impacts on disaster management [40]. For example, Teo found that there were significant variations in disaster preparedness among different ethnicity groups [41]. Cvetković et al. found that men were more prepared than women in flooding events [23]. Although these results are not consistent with our findings, it may be due to the different types of disasters. It is possible that men feel that they are physically stronger and, thus, are more prepared for flooding, while they are less prepared for the pandemic because they may think that if they are infected, they will not get sick. This may be partly why we found that women were more prepared than men in the COVID-19 pandemic. Our finding that there is no impact of ethnicity on COVID-19 awareness and preparedness may be due to the small sample size and that the majority of students were Han.

The findings of this study contribute to the literature and have practical implications. This study is probably the first to look at the effects of anti-epidemic campus signals on students' COVID-19 awareness and preparedness. This study shows how postsecondary institutions' actions can influence awareness and preparedness in the post-COVID-19 era. In addition, it provides further empirical evidence that COVID-19 knowledge can contribute to both awareness and preparedness, and awareness can influence preparedness. Based on these results, we recommend that postsecondary administrators focus on building a tense anti-epidemic atmosphere by establishing more anti-epidemic measures. Students living on campuses without strict anti-epidemic measures may fail to prepare for COVID-19. Once a student is infected, the virus is likely to spread quickly due to the gatherings that occur in campus settings. Thus, it is crucial to increase students' risk perceptions of the pandemic and to be better prepared for future pandemics. Better preparation helps to avoid the kind of losses that occurred at the beginning of 2020. Notably, the findings could also inform policymakers of how to make policy decisions at both the institutional and individual level to better prepare for future pandemics.

The structured questionnaires were carefully designed, and the effect of anti-epidemic campus signals on students' COVID-19 preparedness was comprehensively examined, but this study still has the following limitations. First, there are still unobserved variables, such as the whole nation's anti-epidemic measures, which are also likely to influence the public's preparedness but cannot be directly measured. These unobserved variables are likely to influence the model results but were inevitably tested. Second, psychological variables are very complex, and the study could consider more survey items from multiple aspects. Though we designed our questionnaires comprehensively, it is still possible that other survey items could measure certain latent factor. Third, this study could not draw causal relations between anti-epidemic campus signals and students' preparedness because it is not a fully experimental design. It is still valuable for postsecondary administrators and policymakers to consider that this relationship indeed exists and that corresponding actions can, thus, be taken.

6. Conclusions

Preventing the transmission of COVID-19 is important for education [42]. This study sought to understand the effects of anti-epidemic campus signals on students' COVID-19 preparedness. The results showed positive and significant relationships among these signals, awareness, and preparedness. In addition, we found that students' COVID-19 knowledge can significantly predict their awareness and preparedness, and awareness has a positive association with preparedness. Notably, gender had an influence on students' COVID-19 awareness and preparedness, while ethnicity did not. These findings provide valuable information for postsecondary administrators and policymakers to prepare for future pandemics.

Author Contributions: T.Z. and Q.S. conceptualized the manuscript; Y.Z., C.W. and Q.S. performed data collection and editing; T.Z. took on the leading role in cleaning and analyzing the data and in writing the original draft. All authors have read and agreed to the published version of the manuscript.

Funding: This research was supported by the Zhejiang Province Association of Higher Education Foundation (KT2021394), the National Social Science Foundation of China (20BGL273, BIA190198), the Fundamental Research Fund of the 2021 Provincial Postsecondary Institution, Hangzhou Dianzi University (GK219909299001-242), and the Research Start-up Fund, Hangzhou Dianzi University (KYS265621012).

Institutional Review Board Statement: This study was conducted according to the guidelines of Hangzhou Dianzi University and approved by the Institutional Review Board of Zhejiang Academy of Higher Education.

Informed Consent Statement: Informed consent was obtained from all subjects involved in the study.

Data Availability Statement: According to the data access policies, the data used to support the findings of this study are available from Zhejiang Academy of Higher Education, Hangzhou Dianzi University. Reasonable requests for CSEPPCE data can be made by email: zhaoteng@hdu.edu.cn.

Acknowledgments: The authors would like to thank all the participants of the survey of CSEPPCE.

Conflicts of Interest: The authors declare no conflict of interest.

References

1. Global Map. Available online: https://origin-coronavirus.jhu.edu/map.html (accessed on 6 June 2021).
2. Daniel, S.J. Education and the COVID-19 pandemic. *Prospects* **2020**, *49*, 91–96. [CrossRef]
3. Kumar, R.; O'Malley, P.M.; Johnston, L.D. Association between physical environment of secondary schools and student problem behavior: A national study, 2000–2003. *Environ. Behav.* **2008**, *40*, 455–486. [CrossRef]
4. Weinstein, C.S. Modifying student behavior in an open classroom through changes in the physical design. *Am. Educ. Res. J.* **1977**, *14*, 249–262. [CrossRef]
5. Johnson, S.L. Improving the School Environment to Reduce School Violence: A Review of the Literature. *J. Sch. Health* **2009**, *79*, 451–465. [CrossRef] [PubMed]
6. Tkachuck, M.A.; Schulenberg, S.E.; Lair, E.C. Natural disaster preparedness in college students: Implications for institutions of higher learning. *J. Am. Coll. Health* **2018**, *66*, 269–279. [CrossRef] [PubMed]
7. O'Byrne, L.; Gavin, B.; McNicholas, F. Medical students and COVID-19: The need for pandemic preparedness. *J. Med. Ethics* **2020**, *46*, 623–626. [CrossRef]

8. Stewart, C.R.; Chernoff, K.A.; Wildman, H.F.; Lipner, S.R. Recommendations for medical student preparedness and equity for dermatology residency applications during the COVID-19 pandemic. *J. Am. Acad. Dermatol.* **2020**, *83*, e225–e226. [CrossRef]
9. Hristidis, V.; Chen, S.-C.; Li, T.; Luis, S.; Deng, Y. Survey of data management and analysis in disaster situations. *J. Syst. Softw.* **2010**, *83*, 1701–1714. [CrossRef]
10. Schneider, S.K. *Dealing with Disaster: Public Management in Crisis Situations*; Routledge: New York, NY, USA, 2014.
11. Yu, J.; Sim, T.; Qi, W.; Zhu, Z. Communication with Local Officials, Self-Efficacy, and Individual Disaster Preparedness: A Case Study of Rural Northwestern China. *Sustainability* **2020**, *12*, 5354. [CrossRef]
12. Kohn, S.; Eaton, J.L.; Feroz, S.; Bainbridge, A.A.; Hoolachan, J.; Barnett, D.J. Personal Disaster Preparedness: An Integrative Review of the Literature. *Disaster Med. Public Health Prep.* **2012**, *6*, 217–231. [CrossRef]
13. Hoffmann, R.; Muttarak, R. Learn from the Past, Prepare for the Future: Impacts of Education and Experience on Disaster Preparedness in the Philippines and Thailand. *World Dev.* **2017**, *96*, 32–51. [CrossRef]
14. Thomas, T.N.; Leander-Griffith, M.; Harp, V.; Cioffi, J.P. Influences of Preparedness Knowledge and Beliefs on Household Disaster Preparedness. *Morb. Mortal. Wkly. Rep.* **2015**, *64*, 965–971. [CrossRef]
15. Xu, D.; Peng, L.; Liu, S.; Wang, X. Influences of Risk Perception and Sense of Place on Landslide Disaster Preparedness in Southwestern China. *Int. J. Disaster Risk Sci.* **2018**, *9*, 167–180. [CrossRef]
16. Muzenda-Mudavanhu, C.; Manyena, B.; Collins, A.E. Disaster risk reduction knowledge among children in Muzarabani District, Zimbabwe. *Nat. Hazards* **2016**, *84*, 911–931. [CrossRef]
17. Pinar, A. What is Secondary School Students' Awareness on Disasters? A Case Study. *Rev. Int. Geogr. Educ. Online* **2017**, *7*, 315–331.
18. Johnson, V.A.; Ronan, K.R.; Johnston, D.M.; Peace, R. Evaluations of disaster education programs for children: A methodological review. *Int. J. Disaster Risk Reduct.* **2014**, *9*, 107–123. [CrossRef]
19. Kalanlar, B. Effects of disaster nursing education on nursing students' knowledge and preparedness for disasters. *Int. J. Disaster Risk Reduct.* **2018**, *28*, 475–480. [CrossRef]
20. Ozkazanc, S.; Yuksel, U.D. Evaluation of Disaster Awareness and Sensitivity Level of Higher Education Students. *Procedia-Soc. Behav. Sci.* **2015**, *197*, 745–753. [CrossRef]
21. Eisenman, D.P.; Glik, D.; Gonzalez, L.; Maranon, R.; Zhou, Q.; Tseng, C.-H.; Asch, S.M. Improving Latino Disaster Preparedness Using Social Networks. *Am. J. Prev. Med.* **2009**, *37*, 512–517. [CrossRef]
22. Elliott, J.R.; Pais, J. Race, class, and Hurricane Katrina: Social differences in human responses to disaster. *Soc. Sci. Res.* **2006**, *35*, 295–321. [CrossRef]
23. Cvetković, V.M.; Roder, G.; Öcal, A.; Tarolli, P.; Dragićević, S. The Role of Gender in Preparedness and Response Behaviors towards Flood Risk in Serbia. *Int. J. Environ. Res. Public Health* **2018**, *15*, 2761. [CrossRef]
24. Islam, M.S.; Ullah, M.S.; Paul, A. Community Response to Broadcast Media for Cyclone Warning and Disaster Mitigation: A Perception Study of Coastal People with Special Reference to Meghna Estuary in Bangladesh. *Asian J. Water Environ. Pollut.* **2004**, *1*, 55–64.
25. Takagi, H.; Yi, X.; Fan, J. Public perception of typhoon signals and response in Macau: Did disaster response improve between the 2017 Hato and 2018 Mangkhut typhoons? *Georisk Assess. Manag. Risk Eng. Syst. Geohazards* **2021**, *15*, 76–82. [CrossRef]
26. Ramaprasad, J. Warning Signals, Wind Speeds and What Next: A Pilot Project for Disaster Preparedness among Residents of Central Vietnam's Lagoons. *Soc. Mark. Q.* **2005**, *11*, 41–53. [CrossRef]
27. Duan, T.; Jiang, H.; Deng, X.; Zhang, Q.; Wang, F. Government Intervention, Risk Perception, and the Adoption of Protective Action Recommendations: Evidence from the COVID-19 Prevention and Control Experience of China. *Int. J. Environ. Res. Public Health* **2020**, *17*, 3387. [CrossRef] [PubMed]
28. Bazerman, M.H.; Hoffman, A.J. Sources of Environmentally Destructive Behavior: Individual, Organizational and Institutional Perspectives. *Res. Organ. Behav.* **2000**, *21*, 39–79. [CrossRef]
29. Ikhlaq, A.; Bint-E-Riaz, H.; Bashir, I.; Ijaz, F. Awareness and Attitude of Undergraduate Medical Students towards 2019-novel Corona virus. *Pak. J. Med. Sci.* **2020**, *36*, S32–S36. [PubMed]
30. Ahmed, N.; Shakoor, M.; Vohra, F.; Abduljabbar, T.; Mariam, Q.; Rehman, M.A. Knowledge, Awareness and Practice of Health care Professionals amid SARS-CoV-2, Corona Virus Disease Outbreak. *Pak. J. Med. Sci.* **2020**, *36*, S49–S56. [CrossRef]
31. Anderson, J.C.; Gerbing, D.W. Structural equation modeling in practice: A review and recommended two-step approach. *Psychol. Bull.* **1988**, *103*, 411–423. [CrossRef]
32. Muthén, L.K.; Muthén, B.O. *Mplus User's Guide: Statistical Analysis with Latent Variables, User's Guide*; Muthén & Muthén: Los Angeles, CA, USA, 2017.
33. Muthén, B.; du Toit, S.H.; Spisic, D. *Robust Inference Using Weighted Leastsquares and Quadratic Estimating Equations in Latent Variable Modeling with Categorical and Continuous Outcomes*. 1997. Available online: http://gseis.ucla.edu/faculty/muthen/articles/Article_075.pdf (accessed on 6 June 2021).
34. Hu, L.T.; Bentler, P.M. Cutoff criteria for fit indexes in covariance structure analysis: Conventional criteria versus new alternatives. *Struct. Equ. Modeling A Multidiscip. J.* **1999**, *6*, 1–55. [CrossRef]
35. Jöreskog, K.G. *How Large Can a Standardized Coefficient Be?* 1999. Available online: http://www.ssicentral.com/lisrel/techdocs/HowLargeCanaStandardizedCoefficientbe.pdf (accessed on 6 June 2021).

36. Ruin, I.; Gaillard, J.-C.; Lutoff, C. How to get there? Assessing motorists' flash flood risk perception on daily itineraries. *Environ. Hazards* **2007**, *7*, 235–244. [CrossRef]
37. Cahapay, M.B. Rethinking Education in the New Normal Post-COVID-19 Era: A Curriculum Studies Perspective. *Aquademia* **2020**, *4*, ep20018. [CrossRef]
38. Nindrea, R.D.; Sari, N.P.; Harahap, W.A.; Haryono, S.J.; Kusnanto, H.; Dwiprahasto, I.; Lazuardi, L.; Aryandono, T. Survey data of COVID-19 awareness, knowledge, preparedness and related behaviors among breast cancer patients in Indonesia. *Data Brief* **2020**, *32*, 106145. [CrossRef]
39. Peng, L.; Yang, W.; Zhang, D.; Zhuge, C.; Hong, L. Epidemic analysis of COVID-19 in China by dynamical modeling. *arXiv* **2020**, arXiv:2002.06563.
40. Enarson, E.; Meyreles, L. International perspectives on gender and disaster: Differences and possibilities. *Int. J. Sociol. Soc. Policy* **2004**, *24*, 49–93. [CrossRef]
41. Teo, M.; Goonetilleke, A.; Deilami, K.; Ahankoob, A.; Lawie, M. Engaging residents from different ethnic and language backgrounds in disaster preparedness. *Int. J. Disaster Risk Reduct.* **2019**, *39*, 101245. [CrossRef]
42. Ilyasa, F.; Rahmayanti, H.; Muzani, M.; Ichsan, I.; Suhono, S. Environmental Education for Prevent Disaster: A Survey of Students Knowledge in Beginning New Normal of COVID-19. *Int. J. Adv. Sci. Educ. Relig.* **2020**, *3*, 1–8. [CrossRef]

Assessment of Water Resources Carrying Risk and the Coping Behaviors of the Government and the Public

Ning Zhang, Zichen Wang *, Lan Zhang and Xiao Yang

School of Management, Hangzhou Dianzi University, Hangzhou 310018, China; zhedazhangning@126.com (N.Z.); zhanglan980228@hdu.edu.cn (L.Z.); krisyang@hdu.edu.cn (X.Y.)
* Correspondence: 201030040@hdu.edu.cn; Tel.: +86-17326076166

Abstract: The carrying capacity of water resources is of great significance to economic and social development, eco-environmental protection, and public health. The per capita water resources in Zhejiang Province is only 2280.8 m^3, which is more likely to cause the risk of water resources carrying capacity in the case of water shortage. Therefore, this paper applies Analytic Hierarchy Process-Fuzzy Comprehensive Evaluation and Entropy-Principal Component Analysis to evaluate the vulnerability of disaster-bearers and the risk of disaster-causing factors; it comprehensively evaluates the risk of water resources carrying capacity in Zhejiang Province by constructing risk matrix and ranking scores. The specific results are as follows: According to the comprehensive evaluation of the vulnerability of disaster-bearers in Zhejiang Province from the three aspects of supporting force, regulating force, and pressure, the overall performance was good. In particular, the role of supporting force is the most obvious. In the risk of disaster factors, it was found that industrial structure, climate change, water use efficiency, and population structure have great influence, showing that southern Zhejiang is at a greater risk than northern Zhejiang, and western Zhejiang is at a greater risk than eastern Zhejiang, but the overall score gap is not large. Combining the two results, the order of water resources carrying risk in Zhejiang Province from low to high was Hangzhou, Ningbo, Shaoxing, Jiaxing, Huzhou, Jinhua, Quzhou, Wenzhou, Lishui, Taizhou, and Zhoushan. Finally, according to the development planning of different cities, the coping behaviors of the government and the public regarding water resources carrying risk are put forward.

Keywords: water resources carrying risk; vulnerability of disaster-bearers; hazard of disaster-causing factors; coping behaviors

1. Introduction

The epidemic situation of COVID-19 swept across the world in 2020. In recent years, the number of occurrences and losses caused by both public health events and natural disasters is on the rise [1]. Therefore, the research on public health events, risk assessment of natural disasters, risk management, and other related fields is becoming increasingly intense. China is one of the countries most affected by natural disasters in the world. In order to alleviate the possible impact of disasters and seek the harmonious development of man and nature, it is imperative to carry out natural disaster risk research in China. In 1981, Timmerman formally put forward the concept of vulnerability and applied it to disaster risk assessment [2]. Since then, in the international mainstream research on natural disasters and risks, some scholars have been keen to carry out disaster risk from three aspects: the hazards of disaster-causing factors, the exposure to the disaster-prone environment, and the vulnerability of the disaster-bearers. Additionally, in some studies, exposure to the disaster-prone environment and the vulnerability of the disaster-bearers are summarized as the vulnerability of the disaster-bearing body, and it is pointed out that risk assessment is the basis of risk analysis. As a special natural resource, the lack of effective safety management of water resources leads to many problems, such as flood, drought, water pollution, and water shortage [3]. Furthermore, water resources security risk assessment is an important basis for water resources risk management. China is a water-deficient country, so it is of certain significance to assess the disaster risk caused by water security.

On this basis, scholars have conducted a risk assessment on floods, droughts, water pollution, and water shortage, and have carried out an in-depth study on the factors affecting disaster risk. Most scholars have carried out research on the hazards and vulnerability caused by disasters. Yu pointed out that vulnerability can be defined as the ability of a region to respond to and resist the effects of natural disasters, while risk can be defined as the possibility of natural or man-made physical events, which can show the occurrence of disaster risks in different ways [4]. As far as flood disasters are concerned, Lian took rainfall and tide level as the disaster-causing factors to evaluate the flood and waterlogging risk of coastal cities and found that rainstorms are the main disaster-causing factor in inland areas, and high tide level is the main disaster-causing factor in island areas [5]. Wang assessed the risk of agricultural flooding and waterlogging disasters in Jilin Province and constructed a rainstorm flood risk assessment index system using four aspects: the harmfulness of disaster-causing factors, the sensitivity of disaster-prone environment, the vulnerability of disaster-affected subjects, and the ability of disaster prevention and reduction; it was also pointed out that extreme precipitation events were the main cause of flood disaster [6]. Bouaakkaz assessed the flood disaster in Susi Basin and found that population size, land abuse, overdevelopment, and other factors rapidly aggravated the vulnerability and susceptibility of flood disasters in this area [7]. Lv constructed a comprehensive evaluation index system of urban flood-bearing risk based on the vulnerability of flood-bearing capacity and the vulnerability of disaster prevention and mitigation capacity to study the flood-bearing risk of Zhengzhou and considered that the rapid development of urbanization is the main reason for the increased risk of urban flood and waterlogging disasters [8]. Agrawal studied the relationship between flood risk and resilience in terms of exposure, susceptibility, and lack of coping capacity [9]. Chen studied the mountain torrents in the Guanshan River Basin and found that with the development of the economy and the migration of population, the risk of mountain torrents is increasing [10]. Based on the conclusions drawn by most scholars, it can be found that the influencing factors that cause or destroy the vulnerability of flooding and waterlogging mainly include geography, nature, society, and human behavior, among which human behavior has a greater influence, and the influence caused by a combination of many factors is more serious. For drought disasters, many scholars also assess the risk of drought disasters in terms of hazards, exposure, and vulnerability from different angles. Kim used hydrometeorological and socio-economic data to assess the risk and vulnerability of drought and pointed out that there are both high risk and high vulnerability in high-risk areas [11]. According to the relationship between water use and supply, Wen constructed a set of assessment methods for drought and water shortage risk from the three aspects of the disaster, exposure, and vulnerability, indicating that drought conditions will put additional pressure on the water supply system [12]. Ali believed that drought risk refers to potential disaster losses caused by drought events, which was often described as a function of vulnerability, harmfulness, and exposure, and assessed Africa at the national level, pointing out that controlling population growth has been found to be essential for mitigating drought risk in Africa (or even more effective than mitigating climate change) because it improved socio-economic vulnerability and reduced potential drought risk [13]. In summary, it can be seen that risk assessment from two aspects of risk and vulnerability is a common starting point, which has a longer history of use in the risk research of flood, drought, and other disasters in the field of water resources. Therefore, it can be applied to the risk study of water resources carrying capacity.

Water resources carrying risk is the concrete application of disaster risk theory in the field of water resource carrying capacity [14]. The carrying capacity of water resources was first put forward in the study of the development, utilization, and strategy of water resources in China at the end of the 1980s. Jia defined the carrying capacity of water resources as the maximum supporting capacity of local water resources to the economic development and maintenance of a good ecological environment in a region or river basin under specific development stages and development models [15]. It covered all aspects such as economy, society, resources, and ecological environment [16]. In recent years, many scholars had studied the relationship between water resources carrying capacity and water resources shortage risk [17,18], water resources ecological risk [19,20], water resources security risk [21,22], water resources system risk [23,24], and so on, showing that water resource carrying capacity is closely related to water resources risk. However, as a complex system, the carrying capacity of water resources has the possibility of risk generation. Therefore, based on the theory of disaster risk and the theory of carrying capacity of resources and environment, this paper evaluates the risk of carrying capacity of water resources from the hazards of disaster-causing factors and the vulnerability of disaster-bearers.

The innovation of this paper is that the research on water resources carrying risk in China is still in its infancy, and there is no empirical research on it on the basis of theoretical research; secondly, this paper evaluates the vulnerability of disaster-bearers and the hazards of disaster-causing factors, and then comprehensively obtains the specific situation of water resources carrying risk in Zhejiang Province. The following chapters are as follows: Section 1 is a research design, including concept explanation, index setting, and model construction; Section 2 is a specific empirical analysis of the vulnerability of disaster-bearers and hazards of disaster-causing factors; Section 3 includes conclusions, recommendations, and deficiencies.

2. Research Design

Long defined the risk of water resources carrying capacity as the probability of water resources overloading events under various uncertain situations, and considered that the risk of water resources carrying capacity is closely related to and complementary to the traditional evaluation of water resources carrying capacity, and the former is the extension of the latter, the latter is the basis of the former [14]. From the point of view of disaster risk assessment, the constituent elements of risk mainly include the disaster-causing factors and the disaster-bearers; the regional disaster risk level is affected by the vulnerability of the disaster-bearers and the hazards of disaster-causing factors. According to this, Long summed up the theoretical model of water resources carrying risk, as shown in Figure 1.

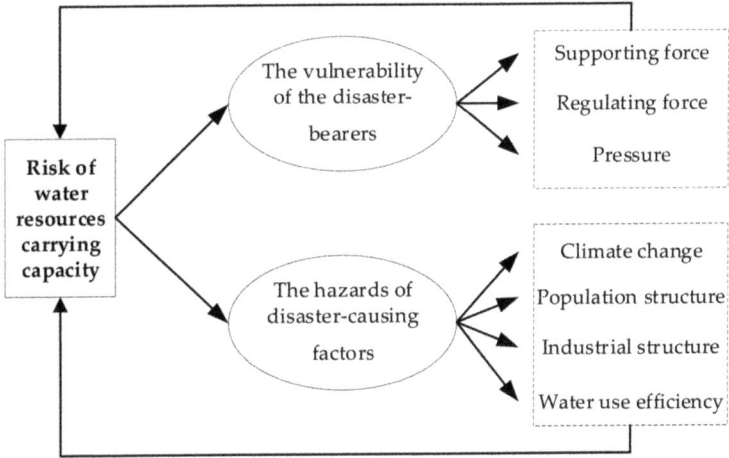

Figure 1. Risk of water resources carrying capacity model.

2.1. The Vulnerability of the Disaster-Bearers

2.1.1. Index Setting

As the research on water resources carrying capacity has become mature in China, and as the basis of water resources carrying risk, academia has a set of relatively rigorous evaluation systems. Therefore, according to the existing mature research, we can summarize a disaster-bearing subject vulnerability index system and its corresponding classification criteria, as shown in Table 1.

Table 1. Index system and grade classification standard of the vulnerability of disaster-bearers.

First-Level Index	Second-Level Index	Type	Grade I (Not Vulnerable)	Grade II (A Little Vulnerable)	Grade III (Vulnerable)
Supporting force	C_1 Per capita water resources (m^3)	P	>1670	1000~1670	<1000
	C_2 Water production modulus (10^4 m^3/km^2)	P	>80	50~80	<50
	C_3 Per capita water supply (m^3)	P	>450	350~450	<350
	C_4 Forest coverage (%)	P	>40	25~40	<25
Regulating force	C_5 Development and utilization of water resources (%)	P	<40	40~70	>70
	C_6 Per capita GDP(Yuan)	P	>24840	6624~24840	<6624
	C_7 Ecological water consumption rate (%)	P	>5	1~5	<1
Pressure	C_8 Per capita domestic water consumption (L)	N	<70	70~180	>180
	C_9 Water consumption of GDP (m^3/10^4 Yuan)	N	<100	100~400	>400
	C_{10} Water consumption of industrial added value (m^3/10^4 Yuan)	N	<50	50~200	>200
	C_{11} Population density (Person/km^2)	N	<200	200~500	>500
	C_{12} Urbanization rate (%)	N	<50	50~80	>80
	C_{13} Farmland irrigation quota (m^3/km^2)	N	<250	250~400	>400

P means positive, N means negative. The calculating methods of each secondary index are shown in Table A1 of Appendix A.

2.1.2. Model Building

As the vulnerability of disaster-bearers has the characteristics of uncertainty and ambiguity, on the basis of referring to the research of other scholars, this paper uses Analytic Hierarchy Process- Fuzzy Comprehensive Evaluation model to evaluate the vulnerability of disaster-bearers regarding water resource carrying risk in Zhejiang Province so as to effectively reflect the results. The Fuzzy Comprehensive Evaluation model is constructed as follows:

Suppose that the two finite field theories are:

$$U = \{U_1, U_2, \cdots, U_n\}, V = \{V_1, V_2, \cdots, V_n\}$$

U represents a set of factors that affect the evaluation object, and V represents a set of comments. $B = A \times E$ represents fuzzy comprehensive evaluation, A represents fuzzy subset on U, $A = \{a_1, a_2, \cdots, a_n\}, 0 \leq a_i \leq 1$, a_i represents the membership degree of U_i to A. It not only represents the role of a single factor U_i in the evaluation factor but also represents the ability of U_i evaluation grade to some extent. $B = \{b_1, b_2, \cdots, b_n\}, 0 \leq b_j \leq 1$, B is the result of the evaluation and is a fuzzy subset on V_j. The membership degree of grade V_j to the fuzzy subset B obtained by comprehensive evaluation is b_j. The evaluation matrix R is:

$$R = \begin{vmatrix} r_{11} & r_{12} & \cdots & r_{1n} \\ r_{21} & r_{22} & \cdots & r_{2n} \\ \vdots & \vdots & \ddots & \vdots \\ r_{n1} & r_{n2} & \cdots & r_{nn} \end{vmatrix}$$

where r_{ij} represents the membership degree of U_i to grade V_j, $r_i = \{r_{i1}, r_{i2}, \cdots, r_{in}\}$ indicates the results of the single factor evaluation of the i factor U_i. The comprehensive evaluation is mainly based on the value of the quantitative evaluation set and the assignment of each grade membership degree in matrix B, and is calculated according to the following formula:

$$a = \frac{\sum_{i=1}^{3} b_i^k a_i}{\sum_{i=1}^{3} b_i^k} \quad (1)$$

In Formula (1), the a value represents the comprehensive score of the vulnerability of the disaster-bearers based on the fuzzy comprehensive evaluation result matrix B. The r_{ij}, in the evaluation matrix R can be compared and analyzed by the actual value of the evaluation factors and the grading index of each evaluation factor, and then the results can be calculated. For grade II, that is, the middle part, the membership degree of the middle point is 1, the membership degree of both edges is 0.5, and the membership degree of the middle point to both sides decreases linearly; for grade I and grade III, the farther away from the critical value, the greater the membership degree of both sides. On the critical value, the membership degree of both sides is 0.5. In order to make the membership function transition smoothly between different levels, it is necessary to fuzzify the membership function. Here, I, II, and III are defined as V_1, V_2, and V_3 respectively.

According to the above assumptions, the calculation formulas of membership functions of each evaluation grade are established. The critical value between grade I and II is expressed by k_1, the critical value between grade II and III is expressed by K_3, and the midpoint value of grade II is expressed by k_2, and $k_2 = (k_1+k_3)/2$. The formula for calculating the membership degree of each evaluation factor to the grade is as follows:

$$U_{V_1} = \begin{cases} 0.5\left(1 + \frac{u_i - k_1}{u_i - k_2}\right), u_i < k_1 \\ 0.5\left(1 - \frac{k_1 - u_i}{k_1 - k_2}\right), k_1 < u_i < k_2 \\ 0, u_i > k_2 \end{cases}, U_{V_2} = \begin{cases} 0.5\left(1 - \frac{u_i - k_1}{u_i - k_2}\right), u_i < k_1 \\ 0.5\left(1 + \frac{k_1 - u_i}{k_1 - k_2}\right), k_1 < u_i < k_2 \\ 0.5\left(1 + \frac{u_i - k_3}{k_2 - k_3}\right), k_1 < u_i < k_2 \\ 0.5\left(1 - \frac{k_3 - u_i}{k_2 - u_i}\right), u_i > k_3 \end{cases}, U_{V_3} = \begin{cases} 0, u_i > k_3 \\ 0.5\left(1 - \frac{u_i - k_3}{k_2 - k_3}\right), k_2 < u_i < k_3 \\ 0.5\left(1 + \frac{k_3 - u_i}{k_2 - u_i}\right), u_i < k_2 \end{cases} \quad (2)$$

Thus, the water resources disaster-bearers matrix R_i, in i City, Zhejiang Province is obtained, and the evaluation value is determined by multiplying the weight matrix obtained by the analytic hierarchy process with the water resources disaster body matrix Ri. Finally, the risk matrix among the first-level indexes is constructed according to the evaluation results, and the vulnerability risk matrix of the final disaster-bearers is formed by pairwise combination.

2.1.3. The Concept and Composition of the Risk Matrix

At the end of the last century, the concept of a risk matrix was first put forward in the United States, and it was initially used to solve risk management problems in the chemical industry and various projects. Subsequently, the risk matrix became widely used in various fields because of its simplicity and intuitive nature. In the risk matrix, the risk criteria are often evaluated by consequences and possibility [25]. When using the risk matrix, deviations can occur when people enter the data, which may lead to different results in the assessment of the same risk [26], and the risk preference cannot be well embedded in the risk matrix [27]. Baybutt believed that in risk management, many scholars use a risk matrix to rate the risk of dangerous scenarios to determine the necessity of risk reduction [28]. An evaluation risk matrix of water resource carrying capacity has been put forward by Jin, in which the pressure, supporting force, and regulating force are regarded as the risk factors affecting water resources carrying capacity [29].

In this paper, based on the risk matrix of water resources carrying capacity, the vulnerability risk matrix of disaster-bearers is further improved. As shown by Table 2, the evaluation grades of row coordinates and column coordinates include grade III, grade II, and grade I, which means vulnerable, a little vulnerable, and not vulnerable, respectively.

eigenvector value = component value/SQR (initial eigenvalue). Thus, the calculation formula of each principal component is as follows:

Where F_{ip} is the score of the p principal component of the i year, λ'_{pj} is the characteristic vector of the j index of the p principal component, and ZX_{ij} is the standardized data of item j of the i year.

3. Entropy Method to Determine the Weight of Each Index

The entropy method determines the weight of each index layer according to the ordered degree of the information contained in each index. The greater the information entropy is, the smaller the index weight is; the smaller the information entropy is, the greater the index weight is. In the process of determining the index weight, the principal component analysis needs the variance contribution rate as the coefficient, including the subjective component, while the entropy method uses the information utility value to determine the index weight, which is an objective weighting method that can avoid the interference of human factors and make the evaluation results more objective.

Define the standardized formula as:

$$f_{ij} = \frac{Y_{ij}}{\sum_{i=1}^{m} Y_{ij}} \tag{6}$$

Then the entropy value and information utility value of each principal component is calculated. The entropy value e of the index j is:

$$e_j = -\frac{1}{\ln m} \sum_{i=1}^{m} f_{ij} \ln f_{ij} \tag{7}$$

The information utility value d of the index j is:

$$d_j = 1 - e_j \tag{8}$$

In determining the entropy weight of each principal component, the greater the information utility value, the greater the entropy weight, indicating that the index is more important. The weight W_j of the j indicator is:

$$W_j = \frac{d_j}{\sum_{i=1}^{p} d_j} \tag{9}$$

4. Evaluation score of the entropy-principal component analysis

Through the analysis of the sample data, the principal component analysis is carried out by using SPSS software, and the principal component score is calculated; the entropy value of each principal component is calculated by using Excel, and the entropy weight of each principal component is obtained, thus Formula (12) is used to calculate the comprehensive score of the hazard index system of disaster-causing factors. The comprehensive score of the i sample is as follows:

$$S_i = \sum_{j=1}^{m} W_j X_{ip} = W_1 X_{i1} + W_2 X_{i2} + \cdots + W_j X_{ip} \tag{10}$$

where S_i is the comprehensive score of the i sample, and X_{ip} is the score of the p principal component of the i sample. The lower the comprehensive score, the lower the risk of disaster factors, the smaller the risk of water resources carrying capacity.

3. Empirical Analysis and Discussion

3.1. Overview of Zhejiang Province

Zhejiang Province is located in the middle and lower reaches of the Yangtze River and borders Shanghai, Jiangsu, Anhui, Fujian, and other provinces. The average precipitation of the whole province in 2019 was 1949.9 mm, which was 18.9% more than that of the previous year and 21.6% more than that of many years. However, the temporal and spatial distribution of precipitation is uneven. The precipitation during the flood season (April to October) accounted for 69.0% of the whole year, generally showing a decreasing trend from west to east and from south to north, and the mountain area is larger than the plain. The coastal mountains are larger than the inland basins. In 2019, the per capita amount of water resources in Zhejiang Province was only 2280.8m^3, which is low when compared globally.

3.2. The Vulnerability of the Disaster-Bearers

3.2.1. Weight Calculation

The vulnerability index data of disaster victims are derived from the Statistical Yearbook of Zhejiang Province in 2020 and the Water Resources Bulletin of Zhejiang Province in 2019. In this paper, the weight of each index is calculated by the AHP method, as shown in Table 4.

Table 4. Weight table of vulnerability indicators for the vulnerability of disaster-bearers.

First-Level Index	Supporting Force				Regulating Force					Pressure			
Second-level index	C_1	C_2	C_3	C_4	C_5	C_6	C_7	C_8	C_9	C_{10}	C_{11}	C_{12}	C_{13}
Weight	0.36	0.21	0.28	0.15	0.43	0.24	0.33	0.26	0.22	0.11	0.17	0.10	0.15

According to Table 4, in the supporting force subsystem, the higher weight indicators are per capita water resources and per capita water supply, both of which are closely related to the total amount of local water resources, that is, the more abundant water resources in a region, the stronger its disaster supporting capacity. Zheng pointed out that water scarcity areas are more likely to face the risk of water resources overload, so it is difficult to provide a guarantee for coordinating the rational utilization of water resources [30]. However, in the regulating force subsystem, the development and utilization rate of water resources and ecological water use rate occupy a higher weight, that is, the higher the eco-environmental quality of an area, the stronger its ability to regulate and control the carrying risk of water resources. Song believed that for different types of water supply and ways of water use, ecological water demand should be ensured as a priority to meet the condition [31]. Planning water consumption quotas and increasing the repetition rate of industrial water use can effectively alleviate the pressure of water shortage. In the pressure subsystem, because the risk pressure of water resources mainly comes from human economic and social activities, the weight gap between each index is not obvious. When studying the carrying capacity of water resources in Jiangsu Province, Li found that promoting water-saving activities and effective sewage discharge can effectively improve the carrying capacity of water resources [32]. At the same time, Tian pointed out that human protection of water resources and social and economic activities have an important impact on the carrying capacity of water resources. Tian also believed that banning sewage discharge and promoting a stricter water resources management system could effectively alleviate the pressure on water resources, thus reduce the cumulative risk of water resources [33].

3.2.2. Calculation of Disaster Bearing Capacity and Construction of a Risk Matrix

According to Formulas (1) and (2), the vulnerability of disaster-bearers in Zhejiang Province is calculated and normalized. The weights of each index of 4 and the results of each index of Table 4 are re-weighted and normalized, and the specific results are shown in Table 5. The results of calculation process are shown in Table A3 of Appendix A.

Table 5. Normalized results of measured values of each subsystem.

City	Supporting Force			Regulating Force			Pressure		
	Grade I	Grade II	Grade III	Grade I	Grade II	Grade III	Grade I	Grade II	Grade III
Hangzhou	0.39	0.45	0.16	0.24	0.35	0.42	0.40	0.33	0.27
Ningbo	0.28	0.48	0.24	0.37	0.24	0.40	0.40	0.32	0.28
Wenzhou	0.30	0.57	0.13	0.28	0.16	0.56	0.14	0.16	0.71
Jiaxing	0.00	0.56	0.44	0.29	0.38	0.33	0.04	0.84	0.12
Huzhou	0.39	0.45	0.16	0.38	0.22	0.40	0.44	0.17	0.39
Shaoxing	0.41	0.43	0.16	0.30	0.27	0.44	0.37	0.31	0.33
Jinhua	0.36	0.49	0.15	0.17	0.19	0.64	0.19	0.27	0.54
Quzhou	0.51	0.34	0.15	0.12	0.31	0.58	0.33	0.24	0.43
Zhoushan	0.12	0.60	0.29	0.41	0.18	0.41	0.08	0.21	0.72
Taizhou	0.36	0.52	0.12	0.18	0.17	0.66	0.16	0.22	0.62
Lishui	0.41	0.36	0.23	0.11	0.28	0.61	0.19	0.22	0.59
Zhejiang	0.43	0.43	0.14	0.16	0.33	0.51	0.32	0.28	0.41

As shown by Tables 4 and 5, because the supporting-regulating forces are positive indicators, the risk grade was determined by the highest value grade, while the supporting-pressure was a negative index, so the risk grade was determined by the lowest value level. For example, Hangzhou had the highest determined value of supporting force grade II, so its determined value is grade II, while the determined value of pressure grade III is the highest, so its fixed value is grade III, and so on. The supporting force, regulating force, and pressure risk grade of each city is obtained, and according to the composition rules of the Table 2 risk matrix, the vulnerability risk matrix of disaster-bearers in Zhejiang Province is obtained, and the specific results are shown in Figure 2.

From Figure 2, it can be seen that for supporting forces, except Quzhou and Lishui, the rest of the cities are grade II. This is because Quzhou and Lishui are located in the southwest of Zhejiang Province, with a large mountain forest area and a small population compared to other cities, so forest coverage, per capita water resources, and water supply will be at a higher level in the province.

As for the regulating force, Zhoushan is a grade I, Jiaxing grade II, and the others are grade III, indicating that the regulating force of most cities in Zhejiang Province is still at a low level. However, it is not difficult to find that the definite values of grade I and grade III in some of these cities are very close, so these cities can make continuous improvements to reduce the development and utilization rate of water resources and ecological water use rate. If we develop the economy on the basis of not destroying water resources, we can better improve the ability to bear and control disasters. However, Quzhou and Lishui, which have excellent performance in supporting force, are in a backward stage, and even the grade I determination value is at a very low level, which may be due to the relatively backward economic development of the two places, and their poor performance in the province due to the low per capita GDP.

In terms of disaster-bearing pressure, it can be seen that southern Zhejiang is obviously better than northern Zhejiang, mainly because a large number of elements in northern Zhejiang continue to be concentrated in the region with the market-oriented reform, which stimulates the expansion of urban land. As a result, the urban development of northern Zhejiang is ahead of southern Zhejiang, highlighting the uneven development. However, the pressure of water resources in a region mainly comes from the population, ecological environment, technology, and economic level. Therefore, when urbanization is not as developed as northern Zhejiang, southern Zhejiang shows less pressure to bear disasters. Hangzhou, Ningbo, Shaoxing, Jiaxing, Taizhou, and other cities are most closely related to the surrounding cities in the industrial economic network pattern. Hangzhou and Shaoxing play an important role in the intermediate transfer and guidance of the province's industrial economy. As a result, these cities are facing greater pressure to bear disasters. However, in the Zhoushan archipelago, due to topography, natural conditions and other reasons, the level of urbanization is not at a high level, so its pressure is naturally small, and its determined value of less than 0.1 is at a higher level. It is very interesting that although Quzhou and Lishui return to grade I again, and the level of industrialization is not high, most of them are extensive, but the gap between them is very obvious. This is because the distribution of industrial enterprises in Quzhou is greater than that in Lishui, for example, Zhejiang Juhua Group is located in Quzhou, while Lishui has few large industrial enterprises, and the government intends to abandon part of its economic development in Lishui to protect the ecological environment.

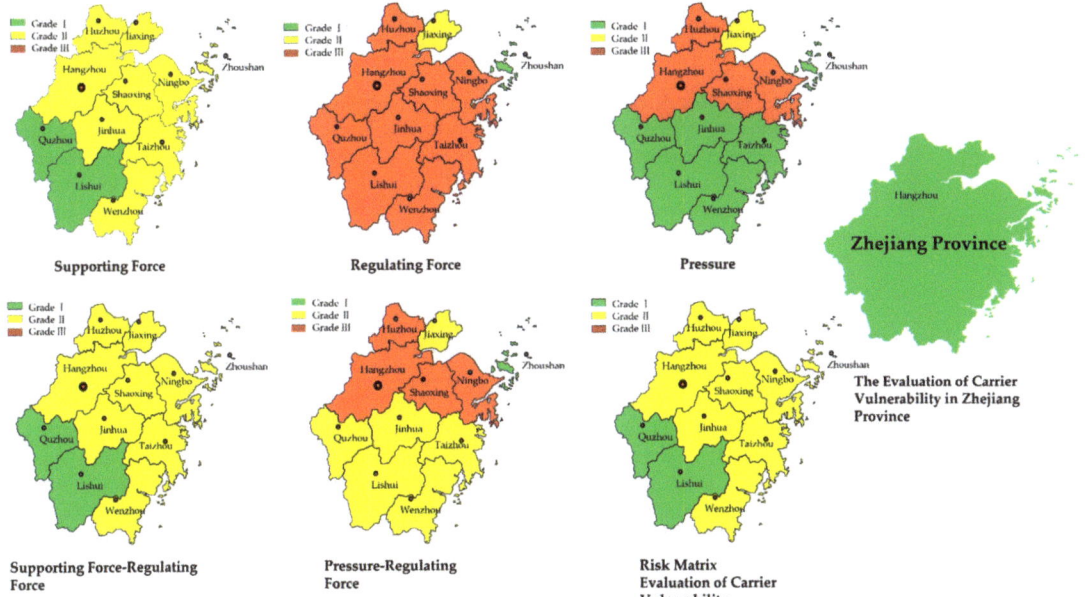

Figure 2. Evaluation grade of the risk matrix for the vulnerability of disaster-bearers in Zhejiang Province.

For the supporting-regulating force composite matrix, we can see that its grade is the same as the supporting force because they are both positive indicators, and there is no resistance to each other; thus, although the regulating force of each city is not good, because the supporting force is enough to cope with the risk of water resources carrying capacity, the primary idea is not to improve the ability to deal with risks by improving the regulation and control ability. However, for the pressure-regulating force, because the pressure is a negative index, there is a relationship between the two, so poor performance in any of them will have an impact on the overall grade. Although the pressure grade of Quzhou, Jinhua, Taizhou, Lishui, and Wenzhou is a grade I, because of their low regulating force, the grade of their composite matrix becomes grade II. This means that it is more likely to face the risk of carrying water resources.

For the final vulnerability of disaster-bearers risk matrix, because the dominance of the supporting-regulating force composite matrix is stronger than that of the pressure-regulating force composite matrix, the final grade of the risk matrix is consistent with the supporting-regulating force composite matrix. We can find that the supporting force plays an important role in the vulnerability of the disaster-bearers. Therefore, each region can give priority to ensuring that the supporting force is at a high grade, and for water-scarce areas, it is necessary to increase water saving and plant drought-tolerant trees so as to gradually increase the amount of water per capita in the future development. For non-water shortage areas, on the basis of water-saving concepts, the most important thing is to further improve the grade of supporting force by increasing forest coverage. Of course, the regulating force is not unimportant because, in most areas of Zhejiang, the subsystem is still at a low level, although it and the supporting force can jointly promote the prevention of water resources carrying risk; however, with the continuous increase in its grade, the pressure-regulating force can also be further enhanced so as to reduce the development pressure of the supporting force. Relatively speaking, the grade of supporting force of various cities in Zhejiang Province is relatively high, and the space for short-term progress is limited. However, there are still gaps in the regulating force that need to be continuously improved.

Finally, for Zhejiang as a whole, the risk matrix synthesis result is independent of the risk matrix synthesis result of each city. The results are a conclusion drawn by calculating the values of Zhejiang Province, using the same matrix judgment and synthesis method. It means that for Zhejiang, without subdividing into subordinate cities, the vulnerability of the disaster-bearers is a grade I, that is, it has a strong ability to cope with the risks carried by water resources. Zhejiang has strong economic strength and attaches great importance to economic development while protecting resources and the environment, paying attention to ecological development. Therefore, Zhejiang is not fragile in the face of water resources carrying risk.

3.3. Hazard of Disaster-Causing Factors

3.3.1. Principal Component Analysis

The index data of hazards of disaster-causing factors are derived from the Statistical Yearbook of Zhejiang Province in 2020 and the Water Resources Bulletin of Zhejiang Province in 2019. According to Formulas (3) and (6), this paper uses SPSS software to analyze the principal components of the data and the results are shown in Tables A4 and A5 of Appendix A. The specific results show that there are five principal components with eigenvalues greater than 1, and the cumulative variance contribution of the first four principal components is 84.955%, close to 85%. Therefore, we can determine that the first four principal components have a great impact on the risk of disaster-causing factors in Zhejiang Province, which is consistent with the number of Table 3 subsystems. There are also more indicators with higher scores of the first principal component, but most of them are concentrated in the industrial structure subsystem, so we determine that the first principal component is divided into the industrial structure subsystem. By analogy, it was concluded that the second principal component is the climate change subsystem; the third principal component is the water use efficiency subsystem, and; the fourth principal component is the population structure subsystem.

3.3.2. Entropy Weight Calculation

According to Formulas (3)–(5) and (7)–(10), the risk entropy, information utility, and weight of disaster-causing factors in Zhejiang Province are calculated, and the specific results are shown in Table 6.

Table 6. Entropy value and weight of each index.

Index	X_{11}	X_{12}	X_{13}	X_{14}	X_{15}	X_{21}	X_{22}	X_{23}	X_{24}	X_{25}
e_j	0.988	0.993	0.992	0.995	0.992	0.994	0.994	0.991	0.989	0.993
d_j	0.012	0.007	0.008	0.005	0.008	0.006	0.006	0.009	0.011	0.007
W_j	7.98%	4.52%	5.05%	3.42%	5.30%	4.23%	4.10%	5.70%	7.33%	4.60%
Index	X_{31}	X_{32}	X_{33}	X_{34}	X_{35}	X_{41}	X_{42}	X_{43}	X_{44}	X_{45}
e_j	0.993	0.991	0.991	0.994	0.994	0.993	0.994	0.991	0.995	0.991
d_j	0.007	0.009	0.009	0.006	0.006	0.007	0.006	0.009	0.005	0.009
W_j	4.69%	6.00%	6.00%	3.96%	4.14%	4.42%	3.61%	5.79%	3.32%	5.82%

From Table 6, we can know that the e_j value of each index is more than 0.9 because the greater the entropy value, the smaller the amount of information and the worse the stability of the system is. Therefore, it can be observed that the degree of disorder of each index is at a high level, indicating that the study of the risk of disaster factors is of significance. Although the overall risk of disaster-causing factors is at a disordered level, there is still a relative gap in the d_j of each index, and the larger the d_j, the greater the impact on the evaluation; thus, the W_j of each index is also different.

3.3.3. Comprehensive Score Calculation of Entropy-Principal Component Analysis

According to Formula (11), and combined with the specific data of Table 6, the comprehensive risk score of disaster-causing factors in Zhejiang Province was calculated and ranked, and the specific results are shown in Table 7.

Table 7. Comprehensive evaluation value of hazard of disaster-causing factors in Zhejiang Province. ($\times 10^{-4}$).

City/Index	X_{11}	X_{12}	X_{13}	X_{14}	X_{15}	X_{21}	X_{22}	X_{23}	X_{24}	X_{25}	X_{31}
Hangzhou	6.13	0.09	2.00	−1.97	5.53	1.60	0.04	0.59	2.08	0.86	2.18
Ningbo	6.72	0.11	2.01	−1.97	4.74	1.34	0.05	0.74	2.63	1.03	2.71
Wenzhou	3.56	0.09	2.12	−2.01	4.93	1.44	0.06	0.57	2.25	0.95	3.54
Jiaxing	7.12	0.08	1.77	−1.04	3.34	1.06	0.07	0.93	2.16	0.62	3.74
Huzhou	7.12	0.07	1.9	−1.88	3.61	1.70	0.07	1.00	3.18	1.13	4.09
Shaoxing	5.54	0.09	1.95	−1.93	4.18	1.61	0.07	0.86	3.56	0.89	3.67
Jinhua	4.35	0.10	2.16	−2.02	4.86	1.71	0.06	0.83	1.78	1.14	3.86
Quzhou	5.14	0.12	2.33	−2.04	4.81	1.98	0.08	1.01	2.59	0.84	4.33
Zhoushan	7.12	0.13	2.22	−2.03	3.09	1.40	0.07	1.13	3.48	1.25	4.36
Taizhou	4.75	0.11	2.23	−2.03	4.99	1.61	0.08	0.74	2.16	1.13	3.77
Lishui	3.56	0.10	3.55	−2.08	6.18	2.11	0.08	1.00	1.91	1.19	4.34
City/Index	X_{32}	X_{33}	X_{34}	X_{35}	X_{41}	X_{42}	X_{43}	X_{44}	X_{45}	Score	Rank
Hangzhou	2.40	2.78	0.14	−3.43	−0.01	2.85	3.15	1.20	−0.73	27.47	1
Ningbo	2.66	3.32	0.25	−3.32	−0.02	2.93	4.85	1.21	−0.82	31.16	5
Wenzhou	4.69	3.68	0.21	−3.40	−0.02	2.70	3.94	1.26	−0.93	29.63	3
Jiaxing	3.50	3.63	0.28	−3.41	−0.02	2.50	3.13	0.69	−1.2	28.95	2
Huzhou	3.79	2.53	0.28	−3.00	−0.03	2.31	3.93	1.09	−1.32	31.55	6
Shaoxing	3.45	4.46	0.25	−3.13	−0.02	2.58	4.32	1.16	−1.15	32.39	8
Jinhua	4.41	3.39	0.20	−3.22	−0.02	2.47	4.87	1.27	−1.18	31.03	4
Quzhou	4.69	4.39	0.22	−2.75	−0.02	1.54	3.24	1.31	−1.42	32.38	7
Zhoushan	3.45	5.06	0.21	−1.72	−0.03	3.07	6.26	1.27	−1.47	38.33	11
Taizhou	4.32	4.79	0.25	−2.76	−0.02	2.63	3.92	1.29	−1.15	32.81	9
Lishui	4.80	4.66	0.21	−2.50	−0.03	2.23	4.16	1.38	−1.42	35.43	10

For the table showing the risk scores of disaster-causing factors, the smaller the score, the smaller the risk, and the higher the ranking. Therefore, from Table 7, it can be seen that the risk of disaster factors in southern Zhejiang is at a greater risk than that in northern Zhejiang and that in western Zhejiang is at a greater risk than that in eastern Zhejiang, but the overall score gap is not large, which is consistent with the results of Shen through the study of water security status and its spatio-temporal variation characteristics in Zhejiang Province. Shen believes that from the spatial level, the spatial heterogeneity of water security in Zhejiang Province is significant, showing the characteristics of "strong in the northeast and weak in the southwest", which is consistent with the pattern of economic and social development of the province; from the level of dynamic change, the regional gap of water security in Zhejiang Province is gradually narrowing, and its optimization speed shows a pattern of "slow in the northeast and fast in the southeast" [34].

As for the industrial structure of the first principal component, the economic level and industrial layout of Zhejiang are stronger in the northeast than in the southwest, and the development level of intelligent industries, green economy, and other emerging fields in Zhejiang cities is also uneven. Additionally, digital economy plays an increasingly important role in the development of China, and it also plays an important role in the field of water resources, such as intelligent water conservancy, intelligent water affairs, intelligent water control, and other related research. Therefore, cities such as Hangzhou, which are leading in the development of the digital economy, have an advantage in this respect.

For the second principal component of climate change, it is not difficult to find that Zhejiang Province has a small area, subtropical monsoon climate, plum rainy season, typhoon season, and other periods, so its precipitation resources are abundant and the climate is appropriate. As a result, the difference between cities is not obvious. Therefore, actively dealing with climate change and preventing global warming can effectively reduce the risk of disaster factors.

As for the water use efficiency of the third principal component, because the main body of water use is small but dense, and the water use behavior is complex, it can be found that the water in the water use efficiency mainly comes from the second principal component and is used in the first principal component, which is dominated by the other two. Therefore, water use efficiency ranks as the third principal component. Extensive and intense human activities will cause serious water environment pollution, which leads to the deterioration of the use of water resources, which not only harms water resources but also becomes a major bottleneck restricting the sustainable development of human society. In 2013, China issued the strictest Water Resources Management system, and at the end of the same year, Zhejiang Province put forward "five-water co-governance", which earlier regulated the water use behavior and effectively improved the water use efficiency; thus, it can be found that the overall performance of Zhejiang Province is better; and there is little difference between cities.

As for the population structure of the fourth principal component, it can be found that the proportion of population density and urban built-up area is relatively high, mainly because the area of Zhejiang Province is small and the level of economic development is high. The continuous increase in the population has led to greater population pressure in limited areas and the expansion of urban areas, thus affecting the ecological environment in many ways, resulting in an increased risk of disaster-causing factors. The disorderly expansion of urban space leads to the destruction of the water circulation system, and the excessive growth of population and the serious lag in the construction of the water supply network and sewage treatment system seriously affect the degree of coordination. Wang also pointed out that measures such as reducing the population growth rate, improving the water use efficiency of the economic system, and optimizing the allocation of water conservancy facilities can effectively improve the carrying capacity of water resources [35]. Therefore, Zhejiang Province should not "change" the economy with people and cities in the process of development, but should comprehensively consider the coordinated development of population, economy, water resources, and other factors so as to reduce the harm of water resources that may be brought in the process of economic construction.

3.4. Risk Assessment of Water Resources Carrying Capacity

The operational Formulas (3)–(5) and (7)–(10) were used to calculate the entropy weight of each subsystem of the vulnerability of disaster-bearers in Zhejiang Province and to rank each subsystem in Table 5 after weighted addition and re-rank the risk of water resources carrying capacity of cities in Zhejiang Province after adding it with the risk ranking of disaster-causing factors in Table 7. The grades from 1 to 11 mean that the vulnerability of the disaster-bearers, the risk of disaster-causing factors, and the carrying risk of water resources all change from small to large, as shown by Figure 3.

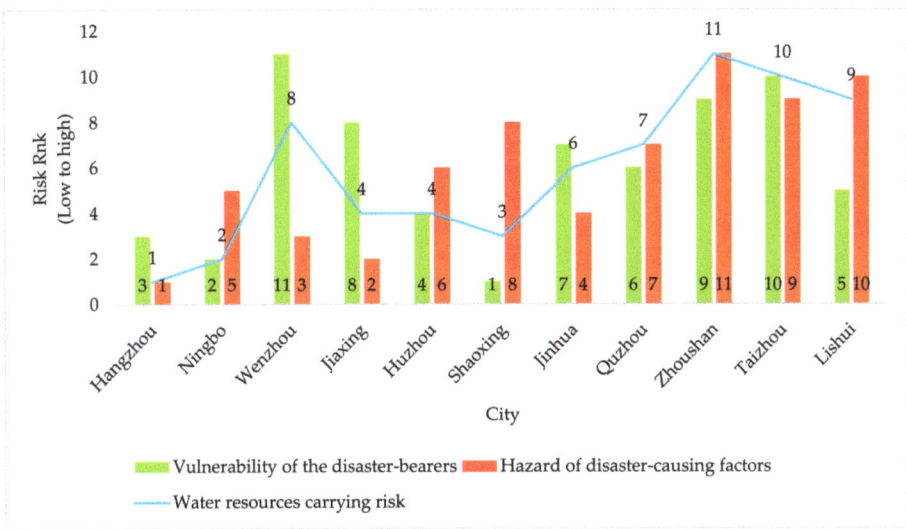

Figure 3. Each city's ranking of vulnerability, hazards, and carrying risks of water resources in Zhejiang Province.

As can be seen from Figure 3, the risk of water resources carrying capacity in economically developed cities such as Hangzhou, Ningbo, and Shaoxing is relatively small, while the relatively less developed cities such as Zhoushan, Lishui, and Quzhou are faced with greater risk of water resources carrying capacity. However, the economic level is not the main factor, such as Wenzhou and Taizhou, their economic level does not belong to the backward position in Zhejiang, but the risk to carrying water resources is still large because they are located in coastal areas and are large cities affected by typhoons. Typhoon transit will have a greater impact on the carrying capacity of local water resources. Typhoons not only cause serious rain and waterlogging, but also have a great impact on economic and social operations. Therefore, the risk to water resources carrying in Wenzhou and Taizhou is not only affected by human activities but also by typhoon-related factors. As far as Wenzhou is concerned, the overall level of Wenzhou is not high because its vulnerability ranks last, which indicates that Wenzhou needs to strengthen the construction of bearing capacity and pay attention to the influence of the risk of disaster-causing factors. As far as Taizhou is concerned, the vulnerability of disaster-bearers and the risk of disaster-causing factors are poor, and the degree of risk to water resources carrying capacity of Taizhou may be higher than that of Zhoushan under the influence of typhoon factors; thus, whether by the water-saving behavior in daily economic activities or the protective behavior in response to typhoons, Taizhou urgently needs to be strengthened, and there is a lot of room for improvement.

For Hangzhou, Ningbo, Shaoxing, and other places, as the urban economic development is relatively high, and the level of investment in water resources management and protection has been in the leading position in the province, which needs to be maintained. One should pay attention to the prevention of non-procedural water resources carrying risks. For Quzhou and Lishui, it can be observed that the vulnerability of the disaster-bearers is in the middle level, but the risk of disaster-causing factors is lower. This is mainly because the eco-environmental level of Quzhou and Lishui is high within the province, which can slightly make up for the deficiency of their vulnerability due to lack of economic development; however, this is not enough to significantly reduce the possibility of water resources carrying risk, resulting in the risk of disaster-causing factors still at a high level, which affects the risk level of water resources carrying capacity.

Finally, as a special island city, Zhoushan Archipelago is affected by many factors, such as geographical environment, economic development, and natural resources. Due to the different geographical characteristics of the islands, there are obvious differences in their industrial structure and the tolerance and coping ability of people in response to natural disasters; the Zhoushan Archipelago area has been prone to storm surges, typhoons, water and other natural disasters since ancient times, so the impact of these on the economic and social life of the island area cannot be ignored. Therefore, in the future, Zhoushan Islands should reasonably control the population, promote technological innovation, improve the efficiency of resource and energy utilization, actively develop the environmental protection industry, and reduce the demand for natural capital. We suggest promoting the coordinated development of human society and the ecosystem so as to reduce the risk of water resources carrying capacity.

4. Deficiency

As a new research field in China, there are still many imperfections in water resources carrying risk assessments, so there are some deficiencies in this study. First of all, this paper directly takes the index system of water resources carrying capacity as the index system of water resources carrying vulnerability, and there may be some indicators that cannot fully explain the concept of "vulnerability", which leads to some deviation in the research. Secondly, the risk matrix grading rules only follow the practice of predecessors and do not change according to the specific research, which may also make the final grading of some cities biased against the real situation. Finally, in the study of the risk of disaster-causing factors, this paper finds that the geographical situation and typhoon climate have an impact on the carrying risk of water resources in an area, but it has not been studied in this paper. Additionally, the specific behavior changes of the government and the public in the face of water resources carrying risk had not been studied in this paper. Therefore, these can be used for future research to continuously improve the risk of water resources carrying capacity.

5. Conclusions

This paper studies the carrying risk of water resources in Zhejiang Province from two aspects: the vulnerability of disaster-bearers and the risk of disaster-causing factors. The Analytic Hierarchy Process-Fuzzy Comprehensive Evaluation method and Entropy-Principal Component Analysis method are used, respectively, for the two aspects, and a risk matrix was constructed for the vulnerability of disaster-bearers. Finally, the ranking and specific conditions of water resources carrying risks of various cities in Zhejiang Province are listed by combining the evaluation results of the two aspects, and the conclusions are as follows.

Zhejiang Province has a strong ability to cope with the water resource carrying risk, but there are still deficiencies in some cities. For the vulnerability of the disaster-bearers, it shows that the northeast region is more vulnerable than the southwest region, and the role of supporting force is more obvious. As for the risk of disaster-causing factors, industrial structure, climate change, water resources utilization efficiency, and population structure have a great impact. The risk of disaster factors in southern Zhejiang is at great risk than that in the north, and western Zhejiang is at a greater risk than that in the east. Generally speaking, Zhejiang Province shows a low risk of carrying water resources in areas with a higher economic level. Therefore, cities in Zhejiang Province can promote energy conservation and emission reduction, encourage water-saving behavior, improve water use efficiency, promote the coordinated development of economy, society, and ecological environment, and reduce the risk of carrying water resources by optimizing the industrial layout and population structure.

To conclude, the risk of carrying capacity of water resources is affected by many aspects, and all of them should be taken into account when preventing the risk. For the government, the most important thing is to measure whether the speed of economic and social development is in line with the state of water resources, whether the development of the economy has caused damage to water resources at the same time; whether water resources are reasonably developed and utilized, and its effective recycling is promoted, and; the government can effectively restrict the behavior of enterprises and the public by promulgating legal provisions. For the public, whether they have water-saving awareness, whether to maintain good daily water-saving behavior and actively participate in water-saving activities are conducive to reducing the risk of water resources carrying capacity.

Author Contributions: Conceptualization, N.Z. and Z.W.; methodology, N.Z. and Z.W.; software, Z.W.; validation, N.Z. and Z.W. and L.Z. and X.Y.; formal analysis, Z.W.; investigation, N.Z. and Z.W.; resources, Z.W.; data curation, Z.W.; writing—original draft preparation, Z.W.; writing—review and editing, N.Z. And Z.W.; visualization, Z.W.; funding Acquisition, N.Z. All authors have read and agreed to the published version of the manuscript.

Funding: This paper was supported by The National Social Science Foundation of China (No. 20BGL188); The Humanities and Social Sciences Foundation of Ministry of Education of China (No.18YJA790107); Natural Science Foundation of Zhejiang Province (No. LY18G030018).

Institutional Review Board Statement: Not applicable.

Informed Consent Statement: "Not applicable" for studies not involving humans.

Data Availability Statement: The data of this paper are derived from the Statistical Yearbook of Zhejiang Province in 2020 and the Water Resources Bulletin of Zhejiang Province in 2019. The link to the Statistical Yearbook of Zhejiang Province in 2020 is http://tjj.zj.gov.cn/flash/tjj/Reports1/2020-%E7%BB%9F%E8%AE%A1%E5%B9%B4%E9%89%B40115/indexcn.html (accessed on 15 April 2021). The link to the Water Resources Bulletin of Zhejiang Province in 2019 is http://www.zjsw.cn/pages/doc.jsp?docId=1658196&catId=1029 (accessed on 15 April 2021). If you are interested in this study and want to obtain the original data, you can contact us.

Conflicts of Interest: The authors declare no conflict of interest.

Appendix A

This is the calculation method of each secondary index in Table 1 of Section 2.1.1, as shown in Table A1.

Table A1. Calculation method of each secondary index in Table 1.

First-Level Index	Second-Level Index	Calculating Method
Supporting force	C_1	Total water resources/Total resident population
	C_2	Total water resources/Regional area
	C_3	Total annual water supply/Total resident population
	C_4	Forest area/Total land area
Regulating force	C_5	Total water supply/Total water resources
	C_6	Total value of GDP/Total population
	C_7	Eco-environmental water consumption/Total water consumption
Pressure	C_8	Total daily water consumption/Total resident population
	C_9	Total socio-economic water consumption/GDP
	C_{10}	Industrial water consumption/Industrial value added
	C_{11}	Resident population/Regional area
	C_{12}	Urban population/total population
	C_{13}	Irrigation water consumption/Irrigation area

This is the calculation method of each secondary index in Table 3 of Section 2.2.1, as shown in Table A2.

Table A2. Calculation method of each secondary index in Table 3.

First-Level Index	Second-Level Index	Calculating Method
Climate change	X_{11}	Σ Monthly average temperature/12
	X_{12}	Σ Monthly average precipitation
	X_{13}	Land income moisture/Ground expenditure water
	X_{14}	Ground expenditure water/Land income moisture
	X_{15}	Total amount of water resources
Population structure	X_{21}	Resident population/Regional area
	X_{22}	Urban population/Total population
	X_{23}	Total resident population
	X_{24}	Natural population growth rate
	X_{25}	Urban area/Regional area
Industrial structure	X_{31}	GDP
	X_{32}	GDP/Total population
	X_{33}	(GDP in this yeay/GDP in last year)-1
	X_{34}	Output value of tertiary industry/Total output value
	X_{35}	Output value of primary industry/Total output value
Water use efficiency	X_{41}	Total industrial water consumption/365
	X_{42}	Total social and economic water consumption/GDP
	X_{43}	Total amount of irrigation water for farmland/Farmland area
	X_{44}	Regional water consumption/Total amount of water resources
	X_{45}	Total domestic water consumption/365

These are data during the calculation process of Table 5 of Section 3.2.2, as shown in Table A3.

Table A3. The results of various indexes shows the vulnerability of disaster-bearers in Zhejiang Province.

Evaluation Index	Zhejiang Province			Hangzhou			Ningbo			Wenzhou			Jiaxing			Huzhou		
	Uv_1	Uv_2	Uv_3	Uv_1	Uv_2	Uv_3	Uv_1	Uv_2	Uv_3	Uv_1	Uv_2	Uv_3	Uv_1	Uv_2	Uv_3	Uv_1	Uv_2	Uv_3
C1	0.43	0.05	0.53	0.28	0.15	0.57	0.11	0.25	0.64	0.13	0.24	0.63	0.00	1.00	0.00	0.22	0.19	0.59
C2	0.25	0.17	0.58	0.28	0.15	0.58	0.22	0.19	0.59	0.38	0.08	0.54	0.00	1.00	0.00	0.12	0.18	0.71
C3	0.00	1.00	0.00	0.00	1.00	0.00	0.00	1.00	0.00	0.00	1.00	0.00	0.00	0.72	0.28	0.04	0.23	0.73
C4	0.40	0.07	0.54	0.42	0.05	0.53	0.34	0.11	0.55	0.41	0.06	0.53	0.00	0.51	0.49	0.34	0.10	0.55
C5	0.37	0.09	0.55	0.37	0.09	0.54	0.37	0.09	0.54	0.38	0.08	0.54	0.01	0.12	0.88	0.34	0.11	0.56
C6	0.46	0.03	0.51	0.48	0.02	0.51	0.47	0.02	0.51	0.44	0.04	0.52	0.47	0.02	0.51	0.46	0.03	0.51
C7	0.00	1.00	0.00	0.00	0.98	0.02	0.00	0.54	0.46	0.33	0.12	0.56	0.00	0.60	0.40	0.00	0.74	0.26
C8	0.00	0.96	0.04	0.00	0.80	0.21	0.00	0.68	0.32	0.00	0.05	0.95	0.00	0.92	0.08	0.00	0.88	0.12
C9	0.28	0.15	0.57	0.29	0.14	0.57	0.29	0.14	0.57	0.29	0.14	0.57	0.28	0.15	0.57	0.27	0.15	0.58
C10	0.08	0.25	0.67	0.20	0.20	0.60	0.24	0.17	0.59	0.12	0.24	0.64	0.20	0.20	0.60	0.21	0.19	0.60
C11	0.00	1.00	0.00	0.00	1.00	0.00	0.00	1.00	0.00	0.00	1.00	0.00	0.00	1.00	0.00	0.00	1.00	0.00
C12	0.00	0.90	0.10	0.00	0.55	0.45	0.00	0.71	0.29	0.00	0.82	0.18	0.00	0.92	0.08	0.00	0.06	0.94
C13	0.02	0.19	0.79	0.00	0.50	0.50	0.19	0.20	0.60	0.00	0.96	0.04	0.00	1.00	0.00	0.00	0.95	0.05

Evaluation index	Shaoxing			Jinhua			Quzhou			Zhoushan			Taizhou			Lishui		
C1	0.28	0.14	0.57	0.40	0.07	0.53	0.48	0.02	0.51	0.00	0.92	0.08	0.39	0.07	0.54	0.49	0.01	0.50
C2	0.28	0.20	0.52	0.25	0.17	0.58	0.39	0.07	0.54	0.00	0.65	0.35	0.31	0.13	0.56	0.38	0.08	0.54
C3	0.00	1.00	0.00	0.00	1.00	0.00	0.32	0.12	0.56	0.00	1.00	0.00	0.00	1.00	0.00	0.00	1.00	0.00
C4	0.39	0.08	0.54	0.41	0.06	0.53	0.43	0.04	0.52	0.36	0.10	0.55	0.41	0.06	0.53	0.45	0.04	0.52
C5	0.36	0.09	0.55	0.38	0.08	0.54	0.39	0.07	0.54	0.38	0.08	0.54	0.39	0.08	0.54	0.40	0.07	0.53
C6	0.47	0.02	0.51	0.45	0.03	0.52	0.44	0.04	0.52	0.47	0.02	0.51	0.45	0.03	0.52	0.44	0.04	0.52
C7	0.00	0.81	0.20	0.24	0.17	0.59	0.00	0.75	0.25	0.00	1.00	0.00	0.33	0.12	0.56	0.00	0.64	0.36
C8	0.00	0.81	0.19	0.00	0.11	0.88	0.07	0.25	0.68	0.00	0.11	0.89	0.00	0.11	0.89	0.05	0.24	0.71
C9	0.28	0.15	0.57	0.28	0.15	0.57	0.24	0.17	0.59	0.30	0.14	0.57	0.28	0.15	0.57	0.27	0.15	0.58
C10	0.16	0.23	0.62	0.00	0.81	0.19	0.00	0.67	0.33	0.00	0.60	0.40	0.14	0.24	0.63	0.16	0.23	0.62
C11	0.00	1.00	0.00	0.00	1.00	0.00	0.12	0.24	0.64	0.00	1.00	0.00	0.00	1.00	0.00	0.28	0.15	0.57
C12	0.00	0.89	0.11	0.00	0.88	0.12	0.05	0.24	0.71	0.00	0.88	0.12	0.01	0.12	0.87	0.01	0.16	0.83
C13	0.05	0.24	0.71	0.14	0.43	0.43	0.00	0.55	0.45	0.37	0.09	0.54	0.00	0.95	0.05	0.02	0.19	0.80

These are the specific results of the principal component analysis in Section 3.3.1, as shown in Tables A4 and A5.

Table A4. Characteristic Root and Cumulative contribution rate of correlation Matrix.

Principal Component	Before Rotation			After Rotation		
	Total	Variance %	Accumulation %	Total	Variance %	Accumulation %
1	7.525	37.627	37.627	6.212	31.060	31.060
2	4.792	23.962	61.589	4.044	20.221	51.280
3	3.486	17.429	79.018	2.932	14.662	65.942
4	1.187	5.937	84.955	2.533	12.663	78.605
5	1.030	5.152	90.107	2.300	11.502	90.107

Table A5. Component score coefficient matrix.

Subsystems	Standardized Index	Component Score			
		1	2	3	4
Climate change	Average air temperature	−0.374	0.766	0.258	0.247
	Average precipitation	−0.513	0.024	−0.496	0.412
	Surface moisture index	−0.695	0.480	0.077	0.082
	Surface drought index	0.458	−0.613	0.470	0.329
	Total amount of water resources	−0.079	0.949	0.133	0.019
Population structure	Population density	0.643	−0.555	−0.217	0.415
	Urbanization rate	0.774	0.214	−0.539	0.018
	Registered population	0.678	0.609	−0.051	0.165
	Natural population growth rate	0.156	0.637	0.392	0.379
	Proportion of urban built-up area	0.613	−0.164	0.546	0.240
Industrial structure	GDP	0.865	0.355	−0.280	−0.034
	GDP per capita	0.702	−0.242	−0.502	−0.170
	The growth rate of GDP	0.712	0.094	0.152	−0.571
	Proportion of tertiary industry	0.063	0.703	−0.367	0.029
	Proportion of primary industry	−0.788	−0.267	−0.475	0.060
Water use efficiency	Industrial water quota	0.883	0.319	−0.006	0.010
	Water consumption of GDP	−0.427	0.099	0.770	−0.232
	Farmland irrigation quota	0.399	0.229	0.790	−0.042
	Development and utilization of water resources	0.575	−0.665	0.395	0.149
	Domestic water quota	0.853	0.421	−0.220	0.044

References

1. Wu, J.R.; Chen, F.; Chen, X.L. Temporal and Spatial Features and Correlation Studies of Global Natural Disasters from 1900 to 2018. *Resour. Environ. Yangtze Basin.* **2021**, *4*, 976–991.
2. Timmerman, P. Vulnerability, resilience and the collapse of society: A review of models and possible climatic applications. Environmental Monograph No. 1, Institute for Environmental Studies, University of Toronto. *J. Climatol* **1981**. [CrossRef]
3. Liang, Y.Y.; Lv, A.F. Risk assessment of water resource security in China. *Resour. Sci.* **2019**, *4*, 775–789.
4. Yu, J.; Kim, J.E.; Lee, J.H.; Kim, T.W. Development of a PCA-Based Vulnerability and Copula-Based Hazard Analysis for Assessing Regional Drought Risk. *KSCE J. Civ. Eng.* **2021**, *25*, 1901–1908. [CrossRef]
5. Lian, J.; Xu, H.; Xu, K.; Ma, C. Optimal management of the flooding risk caused by the joint occurrence of extreme rainfall and high tide level in a coastal city. *Nat. Hazards* **2017**, *89*, 183–200. [CrossRef]
6. Wang, Y.; Liu, G.; Guo, E.; Yun, X. Quantitative Agricultural Flood Risk Assessment Using Vulnerability Surface and Copula Functions. *Water* **2018**, *10*, 1229. [CrossRef]
7. Bouaakkaz, B.; El Morjani, Z.E.A.; Bouchaou, L.; Elhimri, H. Flood risk management in the Souss watershed. *E3S Web Conf.* **2018**, *37*, 04005. [CrossRef]
8. Lv, H.; Guan, X.J.; Meng, Y. Comprehensive evaluation of urban flood-bearing risks based on combined compound fuzzy matter-element and entropy weight model. *Nat. Hazards* **2020**, *103*, 1823–1841. [CrossRef]
9. Agrawal, N.; Elliott, M.; Simonovic, S.P. Risk and Resilience: A Case of Perception versus Reality in Flood Management. *Water* **2020**, *12*, 1254. [CrossRef]

10. Chen, N.; Zhang, Y.; Wu, J.; Dong, W.; Zou, Y.; Xu, X. The Trend in the Risk of Flash Flood Hazards with Regional Development in the Guanshan River Basin, China. *Water* **2020**, *12*, 1815. [CrossRef]
11. Kim, H.; Park, J.; Yoo, J.; Kim, T.W. Assessment of drought hazard, vulnerability, and risk: A case study for administrative districts in South Korea. *J. Hydro Environ. Res.* **2015**, *9*, 28–35. [CrossRef]
12. Wen, L.H.; Shi, Z.H.; Liu, H.Y. Research on risk assessment of natural disaster based on cloud fuzzy clustering algorithm in Taihang Mountain. *J. Intell. Fuzzy Syst.* **2019**, *37*, 1–9. [CrossRef]
13. Ali, A.; Hamid, M.; Andrea, C.; Nicolas, M. Future drought risk in Africa: Integrating vulnerability, climate change, and population growth. *Sci. Total Environ.* **2019**, *662*, 672–686.
14. Long, Q.B.; Zhu, W.B.; Lv, A.F. Theory and methodology analysis for the development of water resources carrying capacity risk monitoring and early warning system. *South North Water Transf. Water Sci. Technol.* **2021**, 1–15.
15. Jia, R.; Xue, H.F.; Xie, J.C.; Jiang, X.H. Research on the Bearing Capacity of Regional Water Resources. *J. Xi'an Univ. Technol.* **1998**, *4*, 54–59.
16. Liu, C.F.; Wang, R.M.; Zhang, X.L.; Cheng, C.L.; Song, H.; Hu, Y. Comparative analysis of water resources carrying capacity based on principal component analysis in Beijing-Tianjin-Hebei region from the perspective of urbanization. *AIP Conf. Proc.* **2017**, *1794*, 030012.
17. Feng, L.H.; Huang, C.F. A Risk Assessment Model of Water Shortage Based on Information Diffusion Technology and its Application in Analyzing Carrying Capacity of Water Resources. *Water Resour. Manag.* **2008**, *22*, 621. [CrossRef]
18. Andrea, B.M.; Tamara, A.; Jochen, S. Risk and sustainability assessment framework for decision support in 'water scarcity—Water reuse' situations. *J. Hydrol.* **2020**, *591*, 125424.
19. Wang, X.K.; Jin, X.L.; Jia, J.J.; Xia, X.M.; Wang, Y.P.; Gao, J.H.; Liu, Y.F. Simulation of water surge processes and analysis of water surge bearing capacity in Boao Bay, Hainan Island, China. *Ocean Eng.* **2016**, *125*, 51–59. [CrossRef]
20. Zhou, X.Y.; Zheng, B.H.; Khu, S.T. Validation of the hypothesis on carrying capacity limits using the water environment carrying capacity. *Sci. Total Environ.* **2019**, *665*, 774–784. [CrossRef]
21. Wolfram, J.; Stehle, S.; Bub, S.; Petschick, L.L.; Schulz, R. Water quality and ecological risks in European surface waters—Monitoring improves while water quality decreases. *Environ. Int.* **2021**, *152*, 106479. [CrossRef]
22. Di, H.; Liu, X.; Zhang, J.; Tong, Z.; Ji, M. The Spatial Distributions and Variations of Water Environmental Risk in Yinma River Basin, China. *Int. J. Environ. Res. Public Health* **2018**, *15*, 521. [CrossRef]
23. Fu, Q.; Gong, F.L.; Jiang, Q.X.; Li, T.X.; Cheng, K.; Dong, H.; Ma, X.S. Risk assessment of the city water resources system based on Pansystems Observation-Control Model of Periphery. *Natural Hazards.* **2014**, *71*, 899–1912. [CrossRef]
24. Meredith, D.; Rebekah, R.B. Transition to a water-cycle city: Sociodemographic influences on Australian urban water practitioners' risk perceptions towards alternative water systems. *Urban Water J.* **2013**, *11*, 444–460.
25. Bao, C.B.; Wu, D.S.; Wan, J.; Li, J.P.; Chen, J.M. Comparison of Different Methods to Design Risk Matrices from the Perspective of Applicability. *Procedia Comput. Sci.* **2017**, *122*, 455–462. [CrossRef]
26. Eric, D.S.; William, T.S.; David, D. Risk matrix input data biases. *Syst. Eng.* **2009**, *12*, 344–360.
27. Thomas, P.; Bratvold, R.B.; Bickel, J.E. The Risk of Using Risk Matrices. *SPE Annu. Tech. Conf. Exhib.* **2014**, *6*, 56–66. [CrossRef]
28. Baybutt, P. Guidelines for designing risk matrices. *Process Saf. Prog.* **2017**, *37*, 49–55. [CrossRef]
29. Wu, C.; Zhou, L.; Jin, J.; Ning, S.; Bai, L. Regional water resource carrying capacity evaluation based on multi-dimensional precondition cloud and risk matrix coupling model. *Sci. Total Environ.* **2020**, *710*, 136324. [CrossRef] [PubMed]
30. Zheng, L.J.; Li, X.P. Evaluation model of regional water resources carrying capacity based on Coordination: A case study of Guangzhou City. *Water Resour. Prot.* **2021**, 1–8.
31. Song, B.; Zhang, F.W.; Yang, H.F.; Liu, C.L.; Meng, R.F.; Nan, T. Source-division evaluation and application on water resources carrying capacity based on ecological priority: Take Baoding Plain, Hebei Province as an example. *Geol. China* **2021**, 1–13.
32. Li, S.P.; Zhao, H.; Wang, F.Q.; Yang, D.M. Evaluation of water resources carrying capacity of Jiangsu Province based on AHP-TOPSIS model. *Water Resour. Prot.* **2021**, *37*, 20–25.
33. Tian, P.; Wang, J.Y.; Hua, W.; Hao, F.H.; Huang, J.W.; Gong, Y.W. Temporal-spatial patterns and coupling coordination degree of water resources carrying capacity of urban agglomeration in the middle reaches of the Yangtze River. *J. Lake Sci.* **2021**, 1–16.
34. Shen, X.M.; Hu, K.L.; Xia, Y.X.; Sheng, Q.; Wang, X.Y. Evaluation on spatio-temporal variation characteristics of water safety in Zhejiang Province. *Yangtze River* **2020**, *51*, 25–30.
35. Wang, L.; Wang, Z.; Liu, X. Water Resources Carrying Capacity Analysis of YarLung Tsangpo River Basin (I). *Water* **2018**, *10*, 1131. [CrossRef]

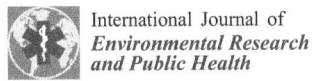

Article

The Factors Affecting Volunteers' Willingness to Participate in Disaster Preparedness

Yingnan Ma [1], Wei Zhu [1], Huan Zhang [2], Pengxia Zhao [1], Yafei Wang [1] and Qiujie Zhang [2,3,*]

[1] Beijing Research Center of Urban Systems Engineering, Beijing 100035, China; yingnanma@126.com (Y.M.); zhuweianquan@126.com (W.Z.); zhaopengxia2021@163.com (P.Z.); yafeiw@126.com (Y.W.)
[2] School of Social Development and Public Policy, Beijing Normal University, Beijing 100875, China; zhanghuan@bnu.edu.cn
[3] Department of Research Project, Beijing Vocational College of Labor and Social Security, Beijing 100029, China
* Correspondence: zhangqiujie@126.com; Tel.: +86-158-0161-1682

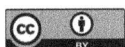

Citation: Ma, Y.; Zhu, W.; Zhang, H.; Zhao, P.; Wang, Y.; Zhang, Q. The Factors Affecting Volunteers' Willingness to Participate in Disaster Preparedness. *Int. J. Environ. Res. Public Health* 2021, *18*, 4141. https://doi.org/10.3390/ijerph18084141

Academic Editors: Yuxiang Hong, Ziqiang Han, Jong-Suk Kim and Joo-Heon Lee

Received: 15 March 2021
Accepted: 12 April 2021
Published: 14 April 2021

Publisher's Note: MDPI stays neutral with regard to jurisdictional claims in published maps and institutional affiliations.

Copyright: © 2021 by the authors. Licensee MDPI, Basel, Switzerland. This article is an open access article distributed under the terms and conditions of the Creative Commons Attribution (CC BY) license (https://creativecommons.org/licenses/by/4.0/).

Abstract: Disaster preparedness is crucial for providing an effective response to, and reducing the possible impacts of, disasters. Although volunteers' participation plays an important role in disaster preparedness, their actual participation in disaster preparedness activities is still low. To find ways to encourage more volunteers to participate, this study analyzed the social background and organizational and attitudinal factors affecting the volunteers' willingness to participate. Questionnaires were distributed to 990 registered disaster volunteers across Beijing and the data were analyzed using linear regression models. Results revealed a weak willingness to participate in disaster preparedness. Only 28.08% of the respondents indicated that they were "very ready" to participate in voluntary disaster preparedness, and 14.65% showed "a little bit" of interest. The following was concluded: (1) Disaster volunteers' social background variables were related to their willingness to participate in disaster preparedness. Compared to male volunteers, female volunteers were more willing to participate. Chinese Communist Party members were more willing to participate than non-members. (2) Providing accidental life insurance for the volunteers had a positive effect on their willingness to participate in disaster preparedness. Provision of more training had a negative effect on the volunteers' willingness to participate, indicating a low quality of training. (3) Organizational identification was positively related to the volunteers' willingness to participate. According to these results, we suggest that volunteer organizations should improve their standards and procedures for disaster volunteer recruitment and selection, and gain a deeper understanding of the needs of the disaster volunteers in order to better motivate them to participate.

Keywords: volunteering; disaster preparedness; accidental life insurance; training; organizational identification

1. Background

Disaster preparedness is a core part of disaster risk management and is crucial for providing an effective response and reducing possible impacts [1]. It is a key indicator of a community's emergency preparedness system vulnerability (EPSV) [2]. Volunteers' participation in disaster preparedness is an effective component of a community's disaster mitigation resources. In the Wenchuan Earthquake in 2008, a variety of people survived because of well-organized disaster relief provided by volunteers. A typical example is provided by the Sang Zao Middle School, where voluntary and regular disaster preparedness activities successfully helped over 2200 faculty and students escape from the school buildings within just two minutes. As a result, not a single person was injured or killed.

The Wenchuan Earthquake marks the start of the Disaster Volunteering Era in China. Since then, disaster preparedness volunteering has been booming, as indicated by the rapidly increasing number of registered disaster volunteers and organizations across the nation. However, the volunteers' actual participation in disaster preparedness activities is not proportionately increasing. A survey from China revealed that as few as one-fourth of the respondents, who were primary care health staff volunteers, participated in emergency response in the past [3]. The same phenomenon was found in other countries as well [4,5]. Why are volunteers reluctant to participate in disaster preparedness? Previous studies have explored the determinants of volunteers' participation in the context of a disaster attack [6], but they have largely ignored disaster preparedness. The current study contributes to the research literature by analyzing the factors affecting volunteers' willingness to participate in disaster preparedness activities. Moreover, the results will help volunteer organization managers improve the standards and procedures of disaster volunteer recruitment and selection, and help them gain a deeper understanding of the needs of the disaster volunteers to better motivate them to participate in disaster preparedness.

In this paper, we explore the current status of volunteers' willingness to participate in disaster preparedness, and then examine the determinants of their willingness to participate. We adopt as our data set a territory-wide survey from Beijing in 2020. Beijing is under constant threat of emerging and re-emerging natural disasters. Located in the North China seismic zone, Beijing is vulnerable to earthquakes. Meanwhile, the rural area of this city, surrounded by the Yan Mountains, faces constant risks of landslides and floods in summer. Thus, voluntary participation in disaster preparedness is very important. There are 140,045 registered disaster volunteers in Beijing, and 71,226 of them belong to 537 volunteer organizations. The organized volunteers are required to provide disaster prevention and mitigation training to local residents, collect and report risk information, and organize regular drills and other disaster preparedness activities for local communities.

This paper is organized as follows. First, the factors affecting volunteers' participation are reviewed and summarized. Second, the data collection procedures, the measurements of variables, and the data analysis methods are presented. Third, the results of regression models are reported. Finally, policy implementation and potential theoretical contributions are discussed.

2. Theoretical Background and Hypothesis Development

A range of explanations have been offered to account for volunteers' participation in disaster response. These can be grouped into three main categories: social background variables, organizational variables, and attitudinal variables.

2.1. Social Background Variables

The relation between social background and volunteers' participation has been discussed relatively thoroughly. The Dominant Status Model of Smith (1994) proposed that people with a higher socioeconomic status are more likely to volunteer [7]. This model has received wide attention [8–12]. Borrowing from this model, Wilson and Musick (1997) established the Resource Model and conceptualized volunteer work as requiring human capital, social capital, and cultural capital [8]. Based on this model, people who have surplus financing and feel secure are more likely to volunteer [13]. Many studies have validated these models, indicating that people with higher education are more likely to volunteer [14,15].

Disaster social science has also borrowed from Liberal Feminist Theory [16]. Disaster organizations often hold the stereotypical notions that women's roles in disaster relief efforts are limited by femininity [16]; however, application studies have revealed complicated results. Some studies have suggested that volunteer participation is greater for males [15,17,18]. Some studies have found that participation can be predicted by a combination of gender and marriage. Andreoni and Payne (2003) found that married males are more sensitive to the price of donating than are married females [19]. Other studies show no significant relationship between gender and volunteering [20]. Moreover, studies on the role of gender in volunteers' participation under disaster scenarios have been quite limited [21]. One survey showed that female healthcare workers are less likely to deploy in the event of a disaster [22].

Political status should also be taken into account. People who are Chinese Communist Party (CCP) members are usually expected to be more devoted to community development; indeed, it has been observed that party members are more willing to volunteer [23].

Based on the analysis above, we propose the following hypotheses:

Hypothesis 1. *Male volunteers are more willing to participate in disaster preparedness.*

Hypothesis 2. *Higher education level has a positive effect on the volunteers' willingness to participate in disaster preparedness.*

Hypothesis 3. *Being a Chinese Communist Party member has a positive effect on the volunteers' willingness to participate in disaster preparedness.*

2.2. Organizational Variables

Volunteering occurs in an organizational context, and thus organizational variables are highly associated with willingness to volunteer [24]. In general, volunteer organizations play a vital role in "pushing" and "pulling" volunteers to participate. On the one hand, a volunteer organization can "push" its members to volunteer by addressing their concerns, such as inadequate capacity and potential physical or mental risks. The Job Demands–Resources (JD-R) model proposes a variety of work-related factors that determine an employee's well-being [25]. Those factors can be categorized as job demands and job resources. Job demands refers to the characteristics of the job that require the employees' physical and/or psychological efforts and cause associated costs. Job resources refer to the characteristics that help reduce job demands and associated costs. Job resources are important in assisting the employees in achieving work goals and fulfilling personal development. For disaster volunteers, participating in disaster preparedness requires professional knowledge and skills and is sometimes risky. Professional knowledge and skills reduce the potential risks and help the volunteers fulfill their tasks [26–28]. Accidental life insurance serves to reduce potential economic loss. From this perspective, disaster volunteer organizations can provide training, guidance, and accidental life insurance to the disaster volunteers and thereby enhance their willingness to participate in disaster preparedness. The positive association between training and people's willingness to volunteer in the event of a disaster has been demonstrated by previous studies [29,30]. However, accidental life insurance has not been taken into account. We interviewed some disaster volunteers, and they all emphasized the importance of accidental life insurance, especially for mountain rescue-related activities.

Based on the analysis above, we propose the following hypotheses:

Hypothesis 4. *Providing accidental life insurance for volunteers has a positive effect on their willingness to participate in disaster preparedness.*

Hypothesis 5. *Providing training for volunteers has a positive effect on their willingness to participate in disaster preparedness.*

Hypothesis 6. *Providing guidance for volunteers has a positive effect on their willingness to participate in disaster preparedness.*

On the other hand, a voluntary organization can "pull" its members to volunteer by providing motivation. Clary and Snyder (1998) proposed Functional Perspective as a way to understand volunteerism [31]. This model assumes that the volunteers' cognitive evaluation of the individual benefits derived from volunteering influence their decision to volunteer. If the volunteers perceive motivational functions in volunteering, they will show more willingness to volunteer. These functions include altruistic tendencies, protecting the self from its negative features, developing one's positive aspects, learning practical knowledge and skills, developing career-related skills, and expanding or maintaining social networks. Positive expectations of behavior have also been found to be important correlates of disaster preparedness [32,33]. Spiritual rewards, such as acknowledgement and encouragement from voluntary organization managers or other volunteers, have a positive effect on the self-efficacy of the volunteers [34]. Developing career-related skills or knowledge can help one to win an advantage in job hunting and/or promotion. In Beijing, volunteers can gain certificates of honor by fulfilling their duties. With these certificates, they can enjoy free access to certain libraries, discounts on haircuts, and other forms of social services. College volunteers with a certificate of honor usually receive extra advantages in scholarship competitions.

Based on the analysis above, we propose the following hypotheses:

Hypothesis 7. *Providing spiritual rewards for volunteers has a positive effect on their willingness to participate in disaster preparedness.*

Hypothesis 8. *Providing certificates of honor for volunteers has a positive effect on their willingness to participate in disaster preparedness.*

2.3. Attitudinal Variables

Social Identity Theory (SIT) proposes that the process of organizational identification helps mediate the interaction between self-interest and the group interest [35]. If the volunteers view the achievements of their organizations as beneficial to themselves, they tend to contribute more effort towards engaging in activities [36].

Based on the analysis above, we propose the following hypothesis:

Hypothesis 9. *Organizational identification has a positive effect on volunteers' willingness to participate in disaster preparedness.*

3. Materials and Methods

3.1. Sampling and Data Collection

The data used in this analysis were collected through the volunteer network of the Beijing Volunteer Association (BVA), founded in 2008, with annual financing from the Beijing local government. Its major responsibilities include the recruitment, selection, training, and deployment of volunteers. All the disaster volunteers (spontaneous volunteers without professional training not included) and organizations in Beijing are registered on its website. At the time of data collection, there were 140,045 registered disaster volunteers, 71,226 of whom belonged to 537 disaster volunteer organizations. BVA extensively collaborates with all levels of government, universities, research institutes, enterprises, communities, and other NGOs. It has established and co-established a number of sites to provide training, drill performance, information collecting, and reporting for the disaster volunteers.

Using a convenience sampling method, 1400 volunteers from 537 disaster volunteer organizations were surveyed online using WeChat (a social media platform used by all registered volunteers) (Tencent, Shenzhen, China). Of these, 990 questionnaires were successfully returned for analysis, giving a response rate of 70.7%. The questionnaire included questions on the social background of the volunteers, basic information on the disaster organization to which they belonged, the job demands and resources provided by the organization, the organizational identification of the volunteers, and the volunteers' willingness to participate in disaster preparedness.

3.2. Measurements

3.2.1. Dependent Variables

Volunteers' willingness to participate in disaster preparedness was measured by a self-reported five-point scale by asking "How much do you want to participate in disaster preparedness-related activities?" Answers were scored on a five-point Likert scale with the following responses: 1 = "Very Much", 2 = "A Little Bit", 3 = "Not Sure", 4 = "Rather Not", and 5 = "Absolutely Not". Questions about the sorts of activities in which volunteers were willing to participate were used as well. The activities mainly included mitigation (e.g., providing information of potential hazards) and capacity building (e.g., providing training for response skills to residents).

The frequency distribution of the dependent variable is shown in Table 1. Overall, 28.08% of the respondents indicated that they were very much ready to participate in voluntary disaster preparedness; 14.65% of the respondents showed a little bit of interest; 31.41% of the respondents answered "Not Sure"; and the rest answered "Rather not" or "Absolutely not".

Table 1. Frequency distribution of the dependent variables (%).

Answers	Willingness to Participate
Very Much	28.08
A Little Bit	14.65
Not Sure	31.41
Rather Not	16.87
Absolutely Not	8.99
Total	100

Figure 1 presents the three major types of disaster preparedness activities the respondents were willing to participate in. It can be seen that the most popular activity was disaster knowledge and skill training (64.7%). Drill organizing ranked second (57.7%). The results reflect a strong need for practical disaster response knowledge and skills.

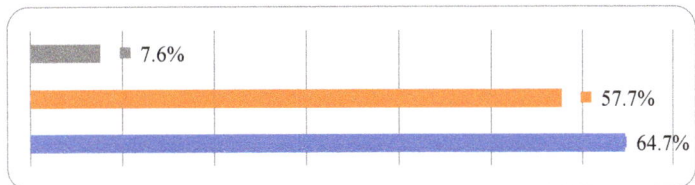

Figure 1. Distribution of willingness to participate in voluntary disaster preparedness activities. Note: Gray bar stands for emergency information report. Orange bar stands for drill organizing activities. Blue bar stands for disaster knowledge and skill training activities.

3.2.2. Independent Variable

There were three sets of independent variables in this analysis. The first set consisted of social background variables, including gender, education, and political status (whether a member of CCP). The detailed distribution of these variables is shown in Table 2.

Table 2. Social background variables of the respondents (%).

Variables	Freq.	Percent	Cum.
Gender			
Female	641	64.75	64.75
Male	349	35.25	100.00
Education			
Middle school and below	17	1.72	1.72
High school	83	8.38	10.10
College and above	890	89.90	100.00
Party			
CCP	412	41.62	41.62
Others	578	58.38	100.00

The second set consisted of organizational variables, which consisted of how often the volunteer organization provided the members with training and guidance to ensure adequate capacity, whether the volunteer organization purchased accidental life insurance for the members to reduce potential risks, and how often voluntary organizations offered spiritual rewards or official certificates of honor for the volunteers. A detailed distribution of the organizational variables is shown in Table 3.

Table 3. Organizational variables of the respondents (%).

Variables	Freq.	Percent	Cum.
Training Provided			
Frequently	341	34.44	34.44
Medium	449	45.35	79.80
Seldom	200	20.20	100.00
Guidance Provided			
Frequently	288	29.09	29.09
Medium	441	44.55	73.64
Seldom	261	26.36	100.0
Accidental Life Insurance Provided			
Yes	443	44.75	44.75
No	547	55.25	100.00
Certification Provided			
Frequently	307	31.01	31.01
Medium	424	42.83	73.84
Seldom	259	26.16	100.0
Spiritual Reward Provided			
Frequently	195	19.70	19.70
Medium	360	36.36	56.06
Seldom	435	43.94	100.0

The third set consisted of attitudinal variables. The organizational identification of the disaster volunteers was measured by a self-reported scale by asking "Do you think becoming a disaster volunteer is your own choice?", "Do you think being a disaster volunteer is important to you?", "Do you care about being a disaster volunteer?", and "Do you think giving up the identity of a disaster volunteer would have a negative impact on you?". These items were scored on a five-point Likert scale: 1 = "Not at all", 2= "Little", 3 = "Hard to say", 4 = "Some", and 5 = "Very much". The mean of the identity degrees was used as the volunteers' willingness predictor (Cronbach's alpha = 0.631). The organizational identification had a mean value of 2.08 with a standard deviation of 0.63, a minimum value of 1, and a maximum value of 4.75 (Table 4).

Table 4. Attitudinal variables of the respondents (%).

Variable	Observation	Mean	SD	Min	Max
Organizational identification	990	2.42	0.50	1	4.75

3.3. Data Analysis Methods

Linear regression models were constructed using willingness to voluntarily participate in disaster preparedness as the dependent variable. The statistical software Stata 15.0 (StataCorp LLC, College Station, TX, USA) was used for data analysis.

4. Results

Table 5 presents the results from the regression analyses. Model 1 only included the social background variables to quantify their influence on willingness to participate. Compared to male volunteers, female volunteers had a stronger willingness to participate in disaster preparedness ($\beta = 0.52$, $p < 0.001$), and thus Hypothesis 1 is rejected. Being a Communist Party member had a positive effect on volunteers' willingness to participate in disaster preparedness ($\beta = -0.22$, $p < 0.05$), and thus Hypothesis 3 is supported. No significant relation was shown between education and willingness to participate and thus Hypothesis 2 is rejected. This may be partly because most of the respondents had received a college degree or above (89.9%).

Table 5. Regression results.

Variables	Model 1	Model 2	Model 3
Gender (Female = 1)	0.52 ***	0.45 ***	0.43 ***
Party (not CCP member = 1)	−0.22 **	−0.22 **	−0.23 **
Education (Middle school and below as reference			
High school	−0.19	−0.21	−0.14
College and above	−0.19	−0.25	−0.19
Accidental Life Provided (Yes = 1)		0.34 ***	0.33 ***
Training Provided (Frequently as reference)			
Medium		−0.02	−0.02
Seldom		0.51	0.46 *
Guidance Provided (Frequently as reference)			
Medium		0.29	0.24
Seldom		0.03	−0.03
Certificates Provided (Frequently as reference)			
Medium		−0.04	−0.07
Seldom		−0.26	−0.28
Spiritual Rewards Provided (Frequently as reference)			
Medium		0.04	−0.01
Seldom		0.05	−0.02
Organizational Identification			0.31 ***
N	990	990	990
R^2	0.15	0.16	0.17

Notes: Standard errors in parentheses. ***, **, and * indicate statistical significance at the 1%, 5%, and 10% levels, respectively.

Model 2 added organizational variables as independent variables. The results show that providing accidental life insurance for the volunteers had a positive effect on willingness to participate ($\beta = 0.34$, $p < 0.001$). This outcome supports Hypothesis 6. Specifically, when other conditions remained unchanged, with accidental life insurance provided by the organization, disaster volunteers' willingness to participate increased by 0.34 units on average. No significant relation was found between training, guidance, certificates, or spiritual rewards and willingness to participate, and thus Hypotheses 5, 6, 7, and 8 are rejected. The effect of gender and political status was still significant, with a minor change in gender.

Model 3 added attitudinal factors as independent variables. The results show that organizational identification was significantly positively related to participation willingness ($\beta = 0.31$, $p < 0.001$), and thus Hypothesis 9 is supported. Specifically, when other conditions remained unchanged, for every one-unit increase in organizational identification of disaster volunteers, their willingness to participate increased by 0.31 units on average. The effects of gender and political status were still significant. The effects of guidance, certificates, or spiritual rewards on willingness to participate were still insignificant. There are two possible explanations for this. One is that the forms and/or content of these measures may not have been sufficiently well designed. Another possible explanation is that guidance, certificates, or spiritual rewards failed to satisfy the actual needs of the volunteers. It is noteworthy that training was partly related to willingness to participate. The outcomes revealed a result opposite to our Hypothesis 5. Provision of training was negatively associated with willingness to participate in disaster preparedness, indicating a low quality of training. More training caused a higher turnover of volunteers.

5. Conclusions

This study aimed to discover the key factors affecting disaster volunteers' willingness to participate in disaster preparedness. Based on prior literature, it categorized these factors into social background, organizational, and attitudinal factors, and it proposed the "pulling" and "pushing" factors of organizations for the first time.

Based on a quantitative survey from 990 registered disaster volunteers across Beijing, we found a weak willingness to participate. Only 28.08% of the respondents indicated that they were "very much" ready to participate in voluntary disaster preparedness, and 14.65% showed "a little bit" of interest. These findings are in agreement with prior studies [3–5,37].

Linear regression models were conducted and the following conclusions were found: (1) Disaster volunteers' social background variables were associated with their willingness to participate in disaster preparedness. Contrary to our hypothesis, female volunteers were more willing to participate in disaster preparedness than male volunteers. It could be inferred that femininity did not limit the females' efforts in disaster preparedness. On the contrary, females may be more caring about the well-being of other people and more devoted to their communities. Being a CCP member was positively associated with the volunteers' willingness to participate in disaster preparedness. As mentioned before, people with traditional virtues, such as being altruistic and devoted to community development, usually have an advantage when applying to become a CCP member. Education had no significant effect on the volunteers' willingness to participate. This may be because most of the respondents of this survey had received a college degree or above (89.9%). (2) Most of the organizational variables were not significantly associated with the volunteers' willingness to participate in disaster preparedness. Among these factors, providing accidental life insurance for the volunteers had a positive effect on their willingness to participate. Provision of accidental life insurance would reduce potential loss for volunteers, as some disaster preparedness activities are risky. Contrary to our hypothesis, provision of training had an opposite effect. This might indicate that a low quality of training caused the turnover of the volunteers. Guidance, certificates, and spiritual rewards had no significant relation to willingness to participate. This indicates the poor quality of the motivating measures or their failure to satisfy the actual needs of the volunteers. (3) Organizational identification was positively associated with the volunteers' willingness to participate and thus supported our hypothesis.

According to the conclusions above, we propose the following suggestions. First, organizations should enroll more CCP members as volunteers, considering their stronger willingness to participate and their commitment to community safety in general. Second, more family support measures should be taken to support female volunteers. Third, all disaster organizations are advised to provide accidental life insurance for volunteers who participate in disaster preparedness. This insurance will provide compensation for potential loss during disaster preparedness activities and thus reduce the safety concerns of the volunteers. Fourth, organizations should pay more attention to culture building. Culture building will enhance organizational identification and thus improve the volunteers' willingness to participate. Last but not least, the quality and content of the training, guidance, certificates, and spiritual rewards provided by the volunteer organizations should be improved. The real motivations behind volunteering should be investigated so that more motivating plans can be made accordingly.

Although this study provides a useful exploration of the correlations between social background, organizational, and attitudinal variables and the volunteers' willingness to participate in disaster preparedness, it has some deficiencies. The findings underscore the importance of social support, such as family support and work unit support. Moreover, the situational variables were not discussed here, which might introduce bias into the results. These supporting factors and situational variables should be taken into account for further investigation. Last but not least, this study adopted a cross-sectional survey data methodology to examine the hypotheses, which limited the assessment of causal inferences [38]. Future studies should use multi-source, multi-level, or longitudinal data.

Author Contributions: The authors' individual contributions are as follows: Q.Z. is in charge of conceptualization, data collection, formal analysis, investigation and writing of the original draft; Y.M. is in charge of funding acquisition, methodology, resources acquisition, software provision, and review and editing; H.Z., W.Z., Y.W., and P.Z. are in charge of project administration, supervision, and validation. All authors have read and agreed to the published version of the manuscript.

Funding: This research was funded by the Project of the National Key Research and Development Program of the 13th Five-Year Plan "Research on Key Technologies of Community Risk Monitoring and Prevention" (2018YFC0809800)" and Beijing Municipal Science and Technology Project "Research and Application of Decision Support Technology Based on Integrated Management of Emergency Plan" (Z181100009018009).

Institutional Review Board Statement: The study was conducted according to the guidelines of the Declaration of Helsinki and approved by the Institutional Review Board of Beijing Research Center of Urban Systems Engineering.

Informed Consent Statement: Informed consent was obtained from all subjects involved in the study.

Data Availability Statement: We signed a non-disclosure agreement with the BVA regarding the data from this survey.

Conflicts of Interest: The authors declare no conflict of interest.

References

1. The International Federation of Red Cross and Red Crescent Societies. Disaster Risk Management Policy. Available online: https://media.ifrc.org/ifrc/wp-content/uploads/sites/5/2020/04/DRM_policy_Final_EN.pdf (accessed on 17 March 2021).
2. Jiang, T. Assessment method of emergency preparedness system vulnerability based on the complex network theory. *J. Risk Anal. Crisis Response* **2012**, *2*, 195–200. [CrossRef]
3. Zhou, Z.; Wang, C.; Wang, J.; Yang, H.; Wang, C.; Liang, W. The knowledge, attitude and behavior about public health emergencies and the response capacity of primary care medical staffs of Guangdong Province, China. *BMC Health Serv. Res.* **2012**, *12*, 338.
4. Levac, J.; Toal-Sullivan, D.; O'Sullivan, T.L. Household Emergency Preparedness: A Literature Review. *J. Community Health* **2012**, *37*, 725–733. [CrossRef] [PubMed]
5. Jones, M.; Berry, Y. Enriching leadership of volunteers in the emergency services. *Aust. J. Emerg. Manag.* **2017**, *32*, 7–8.
6. Hustinx, L.; Cnaan, R.A.; Handy, F. Navigating theories of volunteering: A hybrid map for a complex phenomenon. *J. Theory Soc. Behav.* **2010**, *40*, 410–434. [CrossRef]
7. Smith, D.H. Determinants of voluntary association participation and volunteering: A literature review. *Nonprofit Volunt. Sect. Q.* **1994**, *23*, 243–263. [CrossRef]
8. Wilson, J.; Musick, M. Who cares? Toward an integrated theory of volunteer work. *Am. Sociol. Rev.* **1997**, *62*, 694–713. [CrossRef]
9. Wilson, J. Volunteering. *Annu. Rev. Sociol.* **2000**, *26*, 215–240. [CrossRef]
10. Erdurmazlı, E. Satisfaction and Commitment in Voluntary Organizations: A Cultural Analysis Along with Servant Leadership. *Voluntas* **2019**, *30*, 129–146. [CrossRef]
11. Ackermann, K. Predisposed to Volunteer? Personality Traits and Different Forms of Volunteering. *Nonprofit Volunt. Sect. Q.* **2019**, *48*, 1119–1142. [CrossRef]
12. Ertas, N. How Public, Nonprofit, and Private-Sector Employees Access Volunteer Roles. *J. Nonprofit Public Sect. Mark.* **2020**, *32*, 105–123. [CrossRef]
13. Loseke, D.R. The whole spirit of modern philanthropy: The construction of the idea of charity, 1912–1992. *Soc. Probl.* **1997**, *44*, 425–444. [CrossRef]
14. Sundeen, R.A. Differences in personal goals and attitudes among volunteers. *Nonprofit Volunt. Sect. Q.* **1992**, *21*, 271–291. [CrossRef]
15. Curtis, J.E.; Grabb, E.; Baer, D. Voluntary association membership in fifteen countries: A comparative analysis. *Am. Sociol. Rev.* **1992**, *57*, 139–152. [CrossRef]
16. Phillips, B.D.; Morrow, B.H. *Women and Disasters: From Theory to Practice*; Xlibris: Philadelphia, PA, USA, 2008.
17. Williams, J.A., Jr.; Ortega, S.T. The multidimensionality of joining. *J. Volunt. Action Res.* **1986**, *15*, 35–44. [CrossRef]
18. Palisi, B.J.; Korn, B. National trends in voluntary association membership: 1974–1984. *Nonprofit Volunt. Sect. Q.* **1989**, *18*, 179–190. [CrossRef]
19. Andreoni, J.; Payne, A.A. Do government grants to private charities crowd out giving or fundraising? *Am. Econ. Rev.* **2003**, *93*, 792–812. [CrossRef]
20. Vaillancourt, F.; Payette, M. The supply of volunteer work: The case of Canada. *J. Volunt. Action Res.* **1986**, *15*, 45–56. [CrossRef]
21. Tucker, J.S.; Sinclair, R.R.; Thomas, J.L. The multilevel effects of occupational stressors on soldiers' well-being, organizational attachment, and readiness. *J. Occup. Health Psychol.* **2005**, *10*, 276–299. [CrossRef]

22. Qureshi, K.; Gershon, R.R.; Sherman, M.F.; Straub, T.; Gebbie, E.; McCollum, M.; Erwin, M.J.; Morse, S.S. Health care workers' ability and willingness to report to duty during catastrophic disasters. *J. Urban Health* **2005**, *82*, 378–388. [CrossRef]
23. Li, Q.; Yu, L. Influencing factors and existing problems of volunteering among the youth. *Youth Juv. Res.* **2011**, *2*, 1–5.
24. Penner, L.A. Dispositional and organizational influences on sustained volunteerism: An interactionist perspective. *J. Soc.* **2002**, *58*, 447–467. [CrossRef]
25. Bakker, A.B.; Demerouti, E. The Job Demands-Resources Model: State of the art. *J. Manag. Psychol.* **2007**, *22*, 309–328. [CrossRef]
26. Paek, H.J.; Hilyard, K.; Freimuth, V.; Barge, J.K.; Mindlin, M. Theory-based approaches to understanding public emergency preparedness: Implications for effective health and risk communication. *J. Health Commun.* **2010**, *15*, 428–444. [CrossRef]
27. Adams, R.M.; Karlin, B.; Eisenman, D.P.; Blakley, J.; Glik, D. Who participates in the great ShakeOut? Why audience segmentation is the future of disaster preparedness campaigns. *Int. J. Environ. Res. Public Health* **2017**, *14*, 1407. [CrossRef] [PubMed]
28. Huynh, J.Y.; Xanthopoulou, D.; Winefield, A.H. The Job Demands-Resources Model in emergency service volunteers: Examining the mediating roles of exhaustion, work engagement and organizational connectedness. *Work Stress* **2014**, *28*, 305–322. [CrossRef]
29. Subbarao, I.; Lyznicki, J.M.; Hsu, E.B.; Gebbie, K.M.; Markenson, D.; Barzansky, B.; Armstrong, J.H.; Cassimatis, E.G.; Coule, P.L.; Dallas, C.E.; et al. A consensus-based educational framework and competency set for the discipline of disaster medicine and public health preparedness. *Disaster Med. Public Health Prep.* **2008**, *2*, 57–68. [CrossRef]
30. Damery, S.; Wilson, S.; Draper, H.; Gratus, C.; Greenfield, S.; Ives, J.; Parry, J.; Petts, J.; Sorell, T. Will the NHS continue to function in an influenza pandemic? A survey of healthcare workers in the West Midlands, UK. *BMC Public Health* **2009**, *9*, 142. [CrossRef]
31. Clary, E.G.; Ridge, R.D.; Stukas, A.A.; Snyder, M.; Copeland, J.; Haugen, J.; Miene, P. Understanding and assessing the motivations of volunteers: A functional approach. *J. Personal. Soc. Psychol.* **1998**, *74*, 1516–1530. [CrossRef]
32. Bourque, L.B.; Regan, R.; Kelley, M.M.; Wood, M.M.; Kano, M.; Mileti, D.S. An Examination of the Effect of Perceived Risk on Preparedness Behavior. *Environ. Behav.* **2013**, *45*, 615–649. [CrossRef]
33. Paton, D. Disaster preparedness: A social-cognitive perspective. *Disaster Prev. Manag. Int. J.* **2003**, *12*, 210–216. [CrossRef]
34. Andreoni, J. Impure altruism and donations to public goods: A theory of warm-glow giving. *Econ. J.* **1990**, *100*, 464–477. [CrossRef]
35. Hogg, M.A.; Abrams, D. *Social Identifications: A Social Psychology of Intergroup Relations and Group Processes*; Routledge: London, UK, 1988.
36. Tyler, T.R.; Blader, S.L. The group engagement model: Procedural justice, social identity, and cooperative behavior. *Personal. Soc. Psychol. Rev.* **2003**, *7*, 349–361. [CrossRef] [PubMed]
37. Titko, M.; Ristvej, J.; Zamiar, Z. Population Preparedness for Disasters and Extreme Weather Events as a Predictor of Building a Resilient Society: The Slovak Republic. *Int. J. Environ. Res. Public Health* **2021**, *18*, 2311. [CrossRef] [PubMed]
38. Rubin, A.; Babbie, E.R. *Empowerment Series: Research Methods for Social Work*; Cengage Learning: Stanford, CA, USA, 2016.

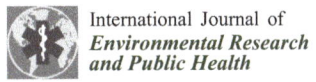

Article

Study on the Formation Mechanism of Medical and Health Organization Staff's Emergency Preparedness Behavioral Intention: From the Perspective of Psychological Capital

Huihui Wang [1], Jiaqing Zhao [2], Ying Wang [3] and Yuxiang Hong [2,*]

1. School of Law and Public Administration, Hunan University of Science and Technology, Xiangtan 411201, China; 1020097@hnust.edu.cn
2. School of Management, Hangzhou Dianzi University, Hangzhou 310018, China; zhaojiaqing@hdu.edu.cn
3. Enze Hospital of Taizhou Enze Medical Center (Group), Taizhou 318050, China; wangy3524@enzemed.com
* Correspondence: hongyx@hdu.edu.cn

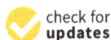

Citation: Wang, H.; Zhao, J.; Wang, Y.; Hong, Y. Study on the Formation Mechanism of Medical and Health Organization Staff's Emergency Preparedness Behavioral Intention: From the Perspective of Psychological Capital. *Int. J. Environ. Res. Public Health* 2021, *18*, 8246. https://doi.org/10.3390/ijerph18168246

Academic Editor: Paul B. Tchounwou

Received: 27 June 2021
Accepted: 31 July 2021
Published: 4 August 2021

Publisher's Note: MDPI stays neutral with regard to jurisdictional claims in published maps and institutional affiliations.

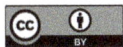

Copyright: © 2021 by the authors. Licensee MDPI, Basel, Switzerland. This article is an open access article distributed under the terms and conditions of the Creative Commons Attribution (CC BY) license (https://creativecommons.org/licenses/by/4.0/).

Abstract: Medical and Health Organization (MHO) staff's emergency preparedness awareness and behaviors are essential variables that affect public health emergency response effectiveness. Based on the theory of psychological capital and the theory of planned behavior (TPB), this study discusses the mechanism of the psychological characteristics of MHO staff on their emergency preparedness behavioral intention (EPBI). To verify the research model, we conducted a web-based questionnaire survey among 243 MHO staff from China and analyzed the data using the structural equation modeling software, AMOS 24.0 (IBM, New York, United States). The empirical results reveal that psychological capital significantly affected cognitive processes theorized by TPB. This study suggests that the positive psychological capital of MHO staff should be developed and managed to improve their EPBI.

Keywords: psychological capital; theory of planned behavior; structural equation model; MHO staff; emergency preparedness behavior

1. Introduction

With deterioration of the natural environment, changes in the international situation, and the acceleration of domestic, economic, and social reform, the frequency of various natural disasters, accident disasters, mass incidents, and public health events has shown a significant upward trend [1–4]. This has become a significant problem affecting economic development, social governance, and even national security. Globally, China is one of the countries with severe disaster risk situations; all types of accidents, hidden dangers and safety risks are prone to occur frequently and continue to evolve into social crises [5]. In particular, the large-scale spread of COVID-19 in the early stage of the pandemic has caused some shortcomings in China's paramount epidemic prevention and control system, public health emergency management system, etc., especially in prevention and early warning, advance disposal, emergency material reserve supply, and other aspects of the lack of necessary adaptability and response [6,7]. Currently, China is in a critical period of moving from a large developing country to a modern social power; the importance and urgency of people's livelihoods and well-being, and social and economic construction, together put forward higher requirements for the national emergency management level [8]. However, the key to excellent emergency management is to strengthen emergency preparedness, which should run through the entire process of dealing with emergencies [7].

Emergency preparedness is a sub-field of emergency management, mainly referring to the establishment and maintenance of various preparations for emergency prevention, early warning, response, and recovery. It includes emergency plan formulation, personnel training, preparation and custody of emergency supplies and equipment, drills within the emergency plan, and connection with external emergency forces. Its ultimate goal is to maintain the emergency capacity and rapid response capacity needed for emergency rescue in relation to significant accidents and ultimately reduce casualties and unnecessary losses [9]. The Medical and Health Organization (MHO) is the main institution for the treatment of diseases and wounds, and its goal is to protect and improve people's health, including hospitals, grass-roots medical and health institutions, professional public health institutions, etc. It is undeniable that no matter what kind of disaster or accident occurs, MHO staff (e.g., doctors, nurses, hospital administrators, CDC staff, health management staff) are at the forefront of response. For example, after an emergency public health incident, the CDC will formulate effective prevention and control measures as soon as possible; the medical and health teams will also go to the disaster areas to assist in medical treatment, health prevention and psychological assistance. As the main force of the rescue effort, they are also the core force in the construction of the national emergency system, and their emergency preparedness capacity and motivation directly affect the quality of medical rescue. Therefore, strengthening the emergency preparedness of MHO staff is also an essential task of national emergency capacity construction [10]. However, currently, few studies have focused on the MHO staff's behavior related to emergency preparedness.

In order to fill the gap in this field, we try to use the theory of planned behavior (TPB) to understand the self-driving mechanism of MHO staff's emergency preparedness behavioral intention (EPBI). In this study, EPBI is considered to be the intention of MHO staff to prepare so as to avoid losses from emergencies. As an essential theory to explain the general decision-making process of individual rational behavior, TPB is widely used in the field of behavioral science, and has been proved to have good explanatory and predictive power of human behavior, and can help researchers understand how people change their behavior patterns [11–13]. TPB holds that thoughtful and planned behavior comes from behavior intention, which depends on people's attitude towards behavior, subjective norms, and perceived behavioral control [14]. However, TPB is not an omnipotent theory, it has a strict scope of application. For example, TPB is based on the premise of completely rational people, and cannot explain well the individual behavior related to emotion and community [15,16]. Therefore, the traditional TPB model is not suitable to predict and explain all behaviors in specific areas, especially those with a wider range, higher conditions, more initiative and beyond the formal requirements of the position. In today's increasingly tricky emergency management situation, the government calls on all MHO staff to be prepared for emergencies, and to respond in order to minimize the damage caused by the accident. These behaviors generally go beyond the job description of MHO employees, and are undertaken entirely out of personal will and have nothing to do with the formal reward system, nor the behavior required by the role. This requires MHO staff to have a broader level of competence, which requires the use a large number of resources that can motivate them to take the initiative to perform a wider range of tasks.

Therefore, we attempt to add psychological capital (PsyCap) as an antecedent factor to the TPB model in order to better understand the formation mechanism of MHO staff's EPBI, and simultaneously stimulate their subjective initiative to participate in emergency preparedness work. The psychological capital proposed by the American management scientist Luthans et al. is regarded as a positive psychological state in the process of individual growth and development, a core psychological element beyond human capital and social capital, and a psychological resource to promote personal growth and performance improvement, including hope, optimism, resilience, and self-efficacy [17–19]. Among these factors, hope refers to "a positive motivational state of success based on the interaction between agents (goal-oriented vitality) and paths (plans to achieve goals)"; optimism is the characteristic of individuals who "expect things to go their way, and generally believe that good, rather than bad, things will happen to them"; resilience is "the positive psychological capacity to rebound, to 'bounce back' from adversity, uncertainty, conflict, failure, or even positive change, progress and increased responsibility"; self-efficacy is a role-breadth characteristic and is defined as an "employee's perceived capability of carrying out a broader and more proactive set of work tasks that extend beyond prescribed technical requirements" [20]. The PsyCap study calls on people to turn their attention to individuals' positive, effective, and efficient aspects, rather than focusing on correcting their problems [21]. Previous studies proved PsyCap to be a kind of psychological quality similar to the state described, and related to specific tasks, situations, and environment; it will change with time and has strong plasticity [22]. More studies support this view, suggesting that PsyCap can be developed through interventions, and influence individual action processes [23–25]. This makes it possible to develop the PsyCap of MHO staff as a positive way to promote their EPBI. Moreover, PsyCap is also regarded as a role-width resource, which is a further expansion and extension of the positive psychological movement in the field of active behavior research, emphasizing the broader role competence of staff members. It helps staff to participate in out-of-role behavior in a more active state. Therefore, this study believes that for the emergency rescue work with MHO staff as the backbone, the positive role that PsyCap can bring is particularly important. It is reasonable for us to explore the intermediary mechanism of TPB in the process of the influence of PsyCap on MHO staff's emergency preparedness behavior.

2. Research Hypotheses and Theoretical Model

2.1. TPB and EPBI

In this study, attitude refers to MHO staff's evaluation of their psychological tendency to conduct emergency preparedness. Perceived behavioral control refers to the difficulty or ease that MHO staff feel when responding to emergency preparedness. Finally, subjective norms refer to the social pressure that MHO staff feel when deciding whether to conduct emergency preparedness, primarily obtained by consulting or observing others' behavior [14].

Firstly, TPB believes that an individual's attitude towards behavior will affect his or her behavioral intention. In a specific time and environment, individuals can acquire a small amount of beliefs about behavior, which are the cognitive and emotional basis of attitude. Among them, individuals with positive beliefs and values about emergency-related content, knowledge, and skills tend to participate in emergency prevention and preparedness, such as emergency knowledge popularization activities and emergency training drills [26]. Those who lack such a good attitude will not continue to conduct the relevant preparatory work [27]. Many previous studies have also confirmed that MHO staff's attitude towards behavior has a positive impact on their behavior intention [28–32]. Therefore, this study infers that a positive emergency attitude indicates a good EPBI. Conversely, a negative attitude reduces an individual's EPBI. Based on the above discussion, this study proposes the following assumption.

Hypothesis 1 (H1). *MHO staff's attitude towards emergency preparedness behavior has a positive impact on their EPBI.*

Secondly, TPB also believes that perceived behavioral control is related to behavior intention. Perceived behavioral control also emphasizes an individual's ability to cope with tasks or make choices to a certain extent, and this ability perception mainly comes from a sense of self-efficacy [33]. Previous studies have shown that self-efficacy is significant in improving levels of responsibility taken in an emergency and work enthusiasm of the MHO staff [34–37]. Among them, MHO staff with high self-efficacy have high expectations of themselves, are more inclined to choose challenging tasks, and will adhere to their behavior even if they encounter difficulties [38–40]. Conversely, individuals with low self-efficacy have low cognition and evaluation of themselves and tend to give up after being negatively affected [41]. Therefore, this study predicts that the stronger the sense of control that MHO staff perceive, the more willing they are to participate in emergency prevention and preparedness. Based on the above discussion, this study proposes the following assumption.

Hypothesis 2 (H2). *MHO staff's perceived behavioral control has a positive impact on their EPBI.*

Finally, an individual's behavior is influenced or motivated by the norms observed in their environment. For example, before the disaster, if the MHO staff noticed that the people around them (superiors, colleagues, and subordinates) were making preventive preparations, they were more likely to participate actively in emergency prevention and preparedness. Conversely, subjective norms also reflect the degree of support of external factors for MHO staff's emergency preparedness behavior to a certain extent and play a vital role in the formation of individual emergency attitudes and perceived behavioral control [42,43]. For example, when MHO staff think that not taking precautions will bring them practical benefits, and the people around them do not show any particular aversion to this behavior, they are likely to treat emergency preparedness with a negative attitude. However, the establishment of appropriate emergency safety education and training mechanisms within the organization can effectively improve MHO staff's working skills and knowledge level and enhance the confidence and determination of internal staff to conduct emergency preparedness. Based on the above discussion, this study proposes the following assumptions:

Hypothesis 3 (H3). *The subjective norms of MHO staff will have a positive impact on their EPBI.*

Hypothesis 4 (H4). *The subjective norms of MHO staff will have a positive impact on their attitude towards emergency preparedness behavior.*

Hypothesis 5 (H5). *The subjective norms of MHO staff will have a positive impact on their perceived behavioral control.*

2.2. PsyCap and TPB

Positive PsyCap reflects the following view: Firstly, regardless of whether they are facing the disaster threat, MHO staff are willing to carry out all kinds of emergency preparedness work [24]. Secondly, MHO staff with high PsyCap expect that emergency preparedness will lead to sound rather than bad results and can maintain this firm belief even if they are affected by adverse events [44]. Thirdly, MHO staff with high PsyCap have confidence in their competence to perform their roles, including emergency preparedness and responses to adverse events and potential threats [21]. Therefore, this study predicts that MHO staff with a higher PsyCap level are more willing to actively participate in emergency preparedness. Based on this, this study proposes the following assumption:

Hypothesis 6 (H6). *MHO staff's PsyCap has a positive impact on their attitude towards emergency preparedness behavior.*

In recent years, through factor analysis, researchers have found that the standard of perceived behavioral control is loaded on two factors. The former reflects the belief in self-efficacy (the individual's judgment of their ability to perform and complete a particular behavior), and the latter reflects the belief in control (the influence of external promotional or hindering factors on the individual's performance of a particular behavior) [45]. However, PsyCap can enhance MHO staff's confidence that they can perform emergency preparedness work and MHO staff's spirit that their emergency preparedness work can effectively reduce the degree of accident damage. Simultaneously, MHO staff with high PsyCap can work efficiently with a positive attitude and pay less attention to adverse problems in their work [46]. Based on the above discussion, this study proposes the following assumption:

Hypothesis 7 (H7). *MHO staff's PsyCap has a positive impact on their perceived behavioral control.*

As an effective way to enhance inner strength and promote individual growth, PsyCap can help MHO staff adjust to psychological and physical problems caused by inter-personal relationships and work stress and improve personal trust and satisfaction [47,48]. Therefore, MHO staff with a high PsyCap level are more willing to believe that their leaders and colleagues attach considerable importance to emergency preparedness. Thus, they also believe that it is imperative to participate in emergency preparedness. Based on the above discussion, this study proposes the following assumption:

Hypothesis 8 (H8). *MHO staff's PsyCap has a positive impact on their subjective norms.*

2.3. The Intermediary Role of Attitude, Perceived Behavioral Control, and Subjective Norms

With careful consideration of Hypothesis 1 to Hypothesis 8, this study puts forward the intermediary hypothesis of attitude, perceived behavioral control, and subjective norms. Based on the previous discussion, this study holds that the positive PsyCap of MHO staff will have a positive impact on their attitude towards emergency preparedness behavior, perceived behavioral control and subjective norms. And these factors will also positively affect their EPBI. Therefore, we have reason to expect that MHO staff's attitude, perceived behavioral control and subjective norms may play an intermediary role between PsyCap and EPBI. In addition, we also believe that MHO employees' subjective norms will promote their attitude and perceived behavioral control, and this study also proposes the intermediary role of attitude and perceived behavioral control between subjective norms and EPBI. The specific assumptions are as follows:

Hypothesis 9 (H9). *The attitude towards emergency preparedness behavior of MHO staff acts as an intermediary between PsyCap and EPBI.*

Hypothesis 10 (H10). *The perceived behavioral control of MHO staff acts as an intermediary between PsyCap and EPBI.*

Hypothesis 11 (H11). *The subjective norms of MHO staff act as intermediaries between PsyCap and EPBI.*

Hypothesis 12 (H12). *The attitude towards emergency preparedness behavior of MHO staff acts as an intermediary between subjective norms and EPBI.*

Hypothesis 13 (H13). *The perceived behavioral control of MHO staff acts as an intermediary between subjective norms and EPBI.*

Figure 1 illustrates the theoretical model.

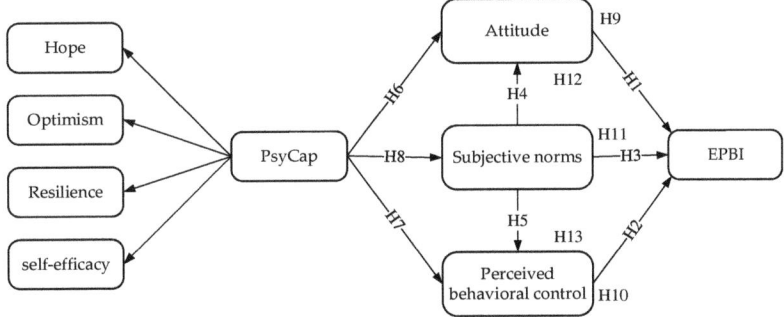

Figure 1. The model of influencing factors of MHO staff's EPBI.

3. Methods

3.1. Study Design

We used the method of questionnaire survey to test the research model. The data sources of this study were accurate and reliable. Firstly, to avoid the systematic error caused by the deviation of the standard method, this study invited five doctoral students of related majors to revise the questionnaire repeatedly to make the question items as concise and easy to understand as possible. To avoid individual repetition, we set the questionnaire to be answered only once per IP address. Secondly, to encourage the participants to answer the questions frankly and truthfully, the online questionnaire used in this study provided complete anonymity—the researchers never knew the identity of the interviewees. Further, the survey was conducted and analyzed outside the organization—enhancing the interviewees' perceived anonymity and actual anonymity. Finally, to ensure the diversity of data sources, this study selected a group of staff composed of staff from different MHOs in China as the research cohort. The use of group samples increases the certainty that the sampling population will accurately represent the target population, and the survey subjects are MHO staff. Therefore, the survey results are more likely to be extended to all MHO workers' groups.

3.2. Measures

The measurement scales used in this study were adapted from the maturity scale proposed by previous scholars. We invited relevant professionals to translate repeatedly to avoid measurement errors caused by semantic differences. Considering that if a potential variable is measured by three or more observation variables, the estimation deviation of the model parameters is almost zero, this study retained three questions for each potential variable. The measurement items of PsyCap were adapted from the questionnaire of Luthans et al. (2007) [49]. The respondents used a 6-point Likert scale to score, ranging from "1 = strongly disagree" to "6 = strongly agree"—the higher the score, the higher the PsyCap level. The measurement items of attitude, subjective norm, and perceived behavioral control were adapted from the questionnaire of Ajzen (2006) [50]. The measurement items of EPBI were adapted from the questionnaires of Miceli et al. (2008) [51], Murphy et al. (2009) [52], Paek et al. (2010) [34] and Hong et al. (2019) [53]. The respondents scored with a 5-point Likert scale, ranging from "1 = strongly disagree" to "5 = strongly agree". The measurement items of each variable are shown in Table 1. In addition, it was considered that the factors that affect individual emergency preparedness behavior were complex and multifaceted, including demographic characteristics, previous disaster experience, etc., [54–56]. Therefore, gender, age, education, occupation, department and experience were selected as control variables in this study.

3.3. Study Participants

Initially, the survey received responses from 289 MHO staff. After excluding incomplete answers and screening out spoiled solutions (for example, the options checked in the whole questionnaire were all the same), it was determined that the number of valid samples was 243, and the effective recovery rate was 84.1%. Among the participants, 80.7% were female, 37.4% were aged between 18 to 24, 72.1% had a Bachelor's degree or above, and 45.7% were nurses. Additionally, 40.7% of the respondents supported Wuhan during the "COVID-19" epidemic. Table 2 shows the demographic characteristics of the participants.

Table 1. Measurement items of latent variables.

Variables	Measurement Items
HP	1. If I should find myself in a jam, I could think of many ways to get out of it. 2. At the present time, I am energetically pursuing my training goals. 3. There are lots of ways around any problem.
OP	1. When things are uncertain for me at work, I usually expect the best. 2. I'm optimistic about what will happen to me in the future as it pertains to work. 3. I approach this job as if "every cloud has a silver lining."
RES	1. When I have a setback at work, I have trouble recovering from it, moving on. 2. I usually take stressful things at work in stride. 3. I feel I can handle many things at a time at work.
SE	1. I feel confident analyzing a long-term problem to find a solution 2. I feel confident in representing my work area in meetings with management. 3. I feel confident contacting people outside my organization (e.g., patients) to discuss problems.
AT	1. I think it is important to participate in emergency preparedness. 2. I think it is beneficial to participate in emergency preparedness. 3. I think it is necessary to participate in emergency preparedness.
SN	1. My families encouraged me to participate in emergency preparedness. 2. My friends encouraged me to participate in emergency preparedness. 3. My managers encouraged me to participate in emergency preparedness.
PBC	1. I have enough skills of emergency preparedness. 2. I have enough knowledge of emergency preparedness. 3. I have sufficient resources for conduct emergency preparedness.
EPBI	1. I will actively participate in the emergency drills in response to major emergencies. 2. I will actively participate in the preparation of public health emergency plans. 3. I will actively popularize the knowledge and skills related to prevention of public health emergencies to the people around me.

Note: HP = hope; OP= optimistic; RES = resilience; SE = self-efficacy; AT = attitude; SN = subjective norms; PBC = perceived behavioral control; EPBI = emergency preparedness behavioral intention.

Table 2. Distribution of demographic characteristics of respondents.

Variables	Classification	Quantity	Percentage
Gender	Male	47	19.3
	Female	196	80.7
Age	18~24	91	37.4
	25~30	29	11.9
	31~40	70	28.8
	41~50	41	16.9
	51~60	12	4.9
Education	Senior high school degree or below	10	4.1
	College degree	58	23.9
	Bachelor degree	152	62.6
	Graduate degree or above	23	9.5
Occupation	Doctor	58	23.9
	Nurse	111	45.7
	The administrative staff of the hospital	12	4.9
	The professional staff of the CDC	1	0.4
	The administrative staff of the CDC	3	1.2
	The administrative staff of other health management departments	15	6.2
Department	Respiratory department	12	4.9
	Infection department	2	0.8
	Critical care department	2	0.8
	Otolaryngology Department	1	0.4
	Operating Room	5	2.1
	Emergency department	4	1.6
	Others	217	89.4
Experience	He/she had the experience of assisting Wuhan during the epidemic	99	40.7
	He/she had no experience of assisting Wuhan during the epidemic	144	59.3

3.4. Data Analysis

In this study, we analyzed the data in three steps. In the first stage, the reliability and validity of the measurement model were tested. In the second stage, the fitness of the structural equation model was tested. In the third stage, the structural equation model was used to test the hypotheses. SPSS 26.0 (IBM, New York, NY, USA) and AMOS 24.0 (IBM, New York, NY, USA) were used to analyze data.

4. Results

4.1. Reliability and Validity Testing

Although all the scales in this study have been recommended, their reliability and validity still need to be evaluated. Firstly, SPSS 26.0 was used to test the reliability of the questionnaire data. The results show that the Cronbach's α coefficient of the whole questionnaire data is 0.960, and that of each variable is more significant than 0.8, indicating that the internal consistency of the scale used in this study is promising.

Secondly, we use AMOS 24.0 software to analyze the validity of the questionnaire data, including the content validity test, convergent validity test, and discriminant validity test. The results show the following: First, except for one observation variable's standard factor load coefficient between 0.6 and 0.7, the other observation variables are all above 0.7; all of them have reached a significant level, indicating that the questionnaire has good content validity. Second, the composite reliability (CR) of each variable is more significant than 0.8, and the average variance extracted (AVE) is more significant than 0.6, indicating that the scale has good convergent validity. Third, there is no obvious distinction between the four substructures of PsyCap, but there is obvious differentiation between these four substructures and other variables, as well as other variables. Previous studies have conceptualized PsyCap into a higher-order structure [49]. Compared with the first-order structure, there are common potential factors among the substructures of the higher-order structure, and there is no need to show discriminant validity [20]. Therefore, the scale in this study has good discriminant validity. In summary, the scale developed in this study has high reliability and validity, and Tables 3 and 4 show the specific analysis results.

Table 3. Analysis of reliability, content validity, and convergent validity of the scale.

Latent Variables	Observation Variables	Mean	SD	Estimate	CR	AVE	Cronbach's α
HP	HP1	4.69	0.848	0.830	0.841	0.638	0.841
	HP2	4.74	0.859	0.807			
	HP3	4.86	0.753	0.758			
OP	OP1	4.71	0.891	0.891	0.921	0.796	0.921
	OP2	4.73	0.891	0.901			
	OP3	4.79	0.852	0.885			
RES	RE1	4.86	0.766	0.746	0.860	0.672	0.849
	RE2	4.51	0.981	0.888			
	RE3	4.47	1.017	0.820			
SE	SE1	4.74	0.819	0.697	0.834	0.628	0.835
	SE2	4.70	0.878	0.830			
	SE3	4.71	0.887	0.842			
AT	AT1	4.33	0.588	0.849	0.931	0.818	0.926
	AT2	4.36	0.589	0.948			
	AT3	4.36	0.610	0.913			
SN	SN1	4.04	0.751	0.859	0.884	0.719	0.874
	SN2	4.07	0.692	0.913			
	SN3	4.19	0.666	0.765			
PBC	PBC1	3.74	0.874	0.821	0.908	0.767	0.903
	PBC2	3.82	0.798	0.864			
	PBC3	3.66	0.877	0.939			
EPBI	EPBI1	4.18	0.674	0.884	0.891	0.732	0.887
	EPBI2	4.18	0.668	0.892			
	EPBI3	4.20	0.700	0.787			

Table 4. Analysis of discriminant validity of the scale.

Variables	HP	OP	RES	SE	AT	SN	PBC	EPBI
HP	0.799							
OP	0.873 ***	0.892						
RES	0.922 ***	0.923 ***	0.820					
SE	0.976 ***	0.814 ***	0.837 ***	0.792				
AT	0.535 ***	0.536 ***	0.445 ***	0.501 ***	0.904			
SN	0.586 ***	0.586 ***	0.562 ***	0.598 ***	0.747 ***	0.848		
PBC	0.578 ***	0.643 ***	0.662 ***	0.594 ***	0.532 ***	0.723 ***	0.876	
EPBI	0.635 ***	0.637 ***	0.570 ***	0.596 ***	0.821 ***	0.650 ***	0.606 ***	0.856

Note: *** $p < 0.001$; The diagonal of the matrix is the square root of the AVE, and below the diagonal is the correlation coefficient between variables.

4.2. Model Fitting

After testing, we found the absolute value of skewness of each observed variable was between 0.155 and 1.140, and the absolute value of kurtosis was between 0.022 and 3.520, so the data formed a normal distribution. The Chi-square versus Mahalanobis distance diagrams of variables were drawn by using the extension program "Normaltest_V1.0" of SPSS 26.0 software. The points in the map approximately formed a straight line, and the combination of all observed variables was close to multivariate normal distribution, so the maximum likelihood estimation method was used to estimate the model parameters. Considering that the overall fitting index value of the model is easily affected by the number of samples, this study selected χ^2/df, RMR, RMSEA, and other indicators to verify the fit of the model and data. The results showed that all the indexes reached or approached the range of recommended standards (χ^2/df = 2.677, RMR = 0.286, RMSEA = 0.083, TLI = 0.867, CFI = 0.880, IFI = 0.881), and there was a good fit between the model and the data. Figure 2 shows the structural model of this study.

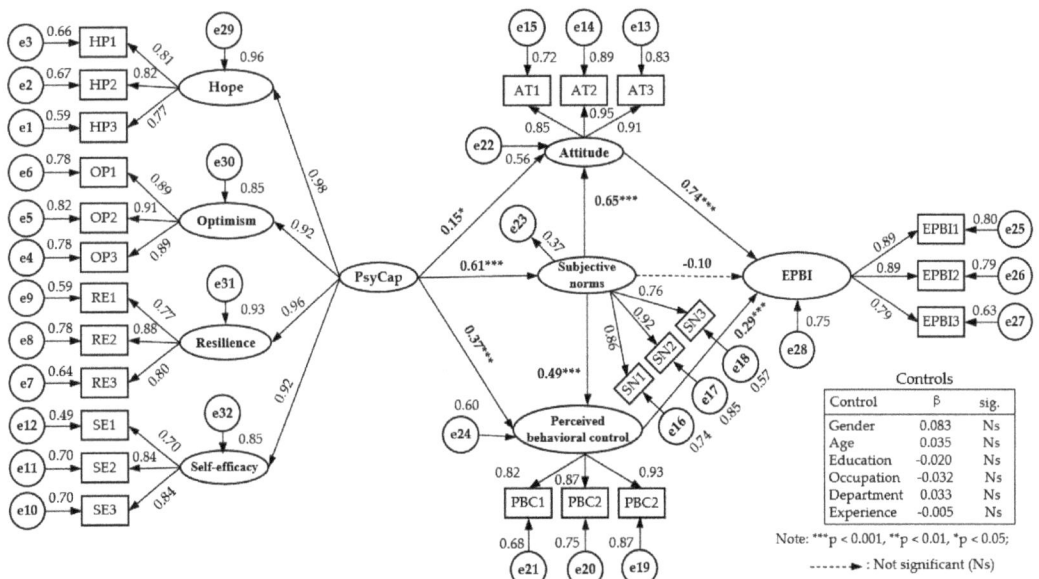

Figure 2. Structural equation model diagram of the influence of PsyCap on EPBI.

4.3. Hypotheses Testing

Based on the premise that the above model fits well, we tested the hypothesis of this study, and Table 5 shows the specific results. Among them, MHO staff's attitude towards emergency preparedness ($\beta = 0.742$, $p < 0.001$) and perceived behavioral control ($\beta = 0.286$, $p < 0.001$) significantly affected their EPBI, supporting Hypothesis 1 and Hypothesis 2. Furthermore, the subjective norms of MHO staff significantly affected their attitude ($\beta = 0.648$, $p < 0.001$) and perceived behavioral control ($\beta = 0.494$, $p < 0.001$), Hypotheses 4 and 5 were supported. Finally, the PsyCap of MHO staff had a significant influence on their attitude towards emergency preparedness behavior ($\beta = 0.152$, $p = 0.022$), perceived behavioral control ($\beta = 0.367$, $p < 0.001$), and subjective norm ($\beta = 0.608$, $p < 0.001$), Hypotheses 6–8 were supported. However, the subjective norms of MHO staff ($\beta = -0.097$, $p = 0.087$) did not significantly impact their EPBI, and Hypothesis 3 was not supported. A reasonable reason for this result may be bias in the study design. For example, there is no unified consensus on the definition of subjective norms in this study. However, this study mainly adopts mandatory subjective norms, whether the essential people around them support their EPBI, but does not consider the demonstrative subjective normative structure, such as how the important people around them do it themselves. Conversely, it may be because most human behaviors are under the control of self-will; thus, the EPBI of MHO staff is more affected by their attitude and perceived sense of behavioral control, making the role of subjective norms relatively weak.

Table 5. Path coefficient estimation and hypothesis test of the model.

Hypotheses	β Coefficient	S.E.	C.R.	p-Value	Is it Established?
Hypothesis 1:AT→EPBI	0.742	0.086	9.481	<0.001	Yes
Hypothesis 2:PBC→EPBI	0.286	0.054	3.934	<0.001	Yes
Hypothesis 3:SN→EPBI	−0.097	0.087	−1.051	0.293	No
Hypothesis 4:SN→AT	0.648	0.064	8.745	<0.001	Yes
Hypothesis 5:SN→PBC	0.494	0.086	7.291	<0.001	Yes
Hypothesis 6:PsyCap→AT	0.152	0.065	2.294	0.022	Yes
Hypothesis 7:PsyCap→PBC	0.367	0.099	5.377	<0.001	Yes
Hypothesis 8:PsyCap→SN	0.608	0.080	8.639	<0.001	Yes

In testing the mediating effect, we consider that the commonly used Sobel method has some limitations. Therefore, this study chooses the bootstrap method to test the mediating role of attitude, perceived behavioral control, and subjective norms in the three paths based on 5000 repeated samplings [57,58]. Table 6 lists specific verification results. Among them, the confidence interval of intermediary pat ① under the Bias-Corrected method at 95% confidence level is [0.005, 0.279], and the p-value is 0.040. The results show that the indirect effect is significant, and its estimated value is 0.122, supporting Hypothesis 9. The confidence interval of intermediary path ② under the Bias-Corrected method at 95% confidence level is [0.024, 0.262], and the p-value is 0.003. The results show that the indirect effect is significant, and its estimated value is 0.113, supporting Hypothesis 10. According to the same method of judgment, we found that paths ④ and ⑤ were also significant, supporting Hypotheses 12 and 13. However, the confidence interval of intermediary path ③ under the Bias-Corrected method at 95% confidence level is [−0.227, 0.076], and the p-value is 0.303. The results show that the indirect effect is not significant, Hypothesis 11 was not supported, echoing the fact that Hypothesis 3 is not valid in the hypothesis test.

Table 6. Test results of mediating effect of the model.

Paths	Indirect Effect	Bias-Corrected			Significance
	Estimate	95%CI		p-Value	
		Lower	Upper		
①PsyCap→AT→EPBI	0.122	0.005	0.279	0.040	Significant
②PsyCap→PBC→EPBI	0.113	0.024	0.262	0.003	Significant
③PsyCap→SN→EPBI	−0.063	−0.227	0.076	0.303	Not significant
④SN→AT→EPBI	0.452	0.310	0.703	<0.001	Significant
⑤SN→PBC→EPBI	0.133	0.055	0.250	0.002	Significant

Note: Lower= lower limit confidence interval; Upper = upper limit confidence interval.

5. Conclusions and Suggestions

With the continuous spread of global social risks, the emergency management system plays an increasingly important role in China's national governance system [59]. However, improving the awareness of MHO staff's emergency preparedness is a crucial way to enhance the foresight, scientificity, and initiative of emergency management. This study focused on the perspective of positive psychological movement and extended the theory of planned behavior by integrating PsyCap to investigate the mechanism by which EPBI is formed. Almost all the hypotheses were supported. The main results of this study are as follows: (1) Attitude and perceived behavioral control had significant positive effects on MHO staff's EPBI, and subjective norms can positively influence attitude and perceived behavioral control. (2) Although subjective norms do not have a direct impact on EPBI, they will have an indirect impact through the intermediary roles of attitude and perceived behavioral control. (3) PsyCap had a significant influence on the decision-making process of MHO staff's emergency preparedness behavior. Specifically, PsyCap had significant positive effects on attitude toward emergency preparedness behavior, subjective norms, and perceived behavioral control. Additionally, PsyCap affected MHO staff's EPBI through the intermediary effects of attitude and perceived behavioral control.

5.1. Theoretical Contribution

Firstly, in the context of China, TPB can be used to predict and explain the intention of emergency preparedness behavior, which further expands the application field of TPB. Secondly, external motivation and internal opportunity work together to affect the EPBI of MHO staff. Most of the previous literature considered the influence of external environmental factors on the formation of EPBI, but seldom considered the influence of individual internal factors. However, the impact of external drivers on EPBI is not real-time and effective, which largely depends on individual self-management. Therefore, this study integrates the theoretical viewpoints in the field of positive psychology and organizational behavior, and further discusses the self-driving mechanism of MHO staff's EPBI. Talking about the influence of PsyCap on EPBI enriches the existing research literature in the field of emergency preparedness, and its conclusions deepen our understanding of the formation mechanism of EPBI. Finally, this study complements the original TPB model by including role-width resources that can promote individuals to perform a broader range of tasks, which provides a more perfect theoretical model for predicting role-width behavior in MHO staff's behavior database and provides an important update consideration for the development of a comprehensive behavioral model.

5.2. Practical Significance

Understanding the influence of TPB on EPBI and the influence of PsyCap on behavioral decision-making process are of great significance to the practical application of positive psychology and organizational behavior theory. Firstly, considering the impact of TPB mechanism on EPBI, management can take corresponding measures to encourage MHO staff to develop the necessary safety skills and knowledge, and stimulate their EPBI in multiple ways. These measures are as follows:

(1) Cultivate crisis awareness and improve the psychological risk reserve of MHO staff.
(2) Strengthen the training of emergency knowledge to make MHO staff fully aware of the significance and value of EP.
(3) Conduct emergency practice drills to enhance the confidence of MHO staff in dealing with unexpected accidents.
(4) Establish emergency logistics support work to ensure MHO workers' health and life safety, etc.

Additionally, the influence of PsyCap on the behavioral decision-making process also provides a unique opportunity for managers to improve the enthusiasm of MHO staff to carry out emergency preparedness work. Managers can develop the PsyCap of MHO staff at the sub-structure or macro-level to improve their attitude towards emergency preparedness behavior, perceived behavioral control and subjective norms. The following are several measures to develop the PsyCap of MHO staff:

(1) Involve MHO staff in the process of preparing emergency preparedness and response plans.
(2) Make realistic and optimistic expectations to counteract the pessimism of MHO staff about emergency preparedness.
(3) Reinforce the transferable value of emergency preparation behavior in the career development of MHO staff.
(4) Provide positive feedback to MHO staff who are actively involved in emergency preparedness, etc.

5.3. Limitations and Prospect

This study has important theoretical and practical significance for understanding and stimulating MHO staff's EPBI, but there are still some limitations. First, the subjects of this study are MHO staff, and the original data were collected through the form of a network questionnaire; hence, the homologous bias cannot be eliminated. Therefore, the research method should be further improved in subsequent studies. Second, the model in this study only considered the mediating effect and did not involve moderating variables. Therefore, future studies should consider more influencing variables to make the results more objective and comprehensive. Finally, the samples used in this study to verify the hypothesis are from China, and whether the research results can be inferred in other countries (regions) needs to be further verified. Follow-up research can increase the scope of the survey and sample size, so that the research results can adapt to a wider range of research objects, and improve the external validity of the research results.

Author Contributions: Conceptualization, Y.H.; methodology, Y.H. and J.Z.; investigation, H.W., Y.W., Y.H.; writing—original draft preparation, J.Z. and Y.H.; writing—review and editing, Y.H. and H.W.; funding acquisition, H.W. and Y.H. All authors have read and agreed to the published version of the manuscript.

Funding: This research was funded by Hunan Provincial Philosophy and Social Sciences Planning Project of China (20YBA113) and Zhejiang Provincial Philosophy and Social Sciences Planning Project of China (20NDQN285YB).

Institutional Review Board Statement: Not applicable.

Informed Consent Statement: Not applicable.

Conflicts of Interest: The authors declare no conflict of interest.

References

1. Pu, C.Y.; Liu, Z.; Pan, X.J.; Addai, B. The impact of natural disasters on China's macro economy. *Environ. Sci. Pollut. Res.* **2020**, *27*, 43987–43998. [CrossRef]
2. Xiao, W.; Xu, J.F.; Lv, X.J. Establishing a georeferenced spatio-temporal database for Chinese coal mining accidents between 2000 and 2015. *Geomat. Nat. Hazards Risk* **2019**, *10*, 242–270. [CrossRef]
3. Zha, D.J. Non-Traditional Security and China-US Relations. *Asian Perspect.* **2021**, *45*, 75–81.
4. Si, R.S.; Lu, Q.; Aziz, N. Impact of COVID-19 on peoples' willingness to consume wild animals: Empirical insights from China. *One Health* **2021**, *12*, 100240. [CrossRef]
5. Wu, Q.; Han, J.W.; Lei, C.Q.; Ding, W.; Li, B.; Zhang, L. The challenges and countermeasures in emergency management after the establishment of the ministry of emergency management of China: A case study. *Int. J. Disaster Risk Reduct.* **2021**, *55*, 102075. [CrossRef]
6. Cao, Y.L.; Shan, J.; Gong, Z.Z.; Kuang, J.Q.; Gao, Y. Status and Challenges of Public Health Emergency Management in China Related to COVID-19. *Front. Public Health* **2020**, *8*, 250. [CrossRef]
7. Kong, F.; Sun, S. Understanding and Strengthening the Emergency Management and Comprehensive Disaster Reduction in China's Rural Areas: Lessons from Coping with the COVID-19 Epidemic. *Sustainability* **2021**, *13*, 3642. [CrossRef]
8. Luo, H.S.; Qian, H.W. Research on the basic theory and practice of emergency management in China in the new development stage. *China Emerg. Manag.* **2021**, *4*, 18–29.
9. Day, A.; Staniszewska, S.; Bullock, I. Planning for Chaos: Developing the Concept of Emergency Preparedness through the Experience of the Paramedic. *J. Emerg. Nurs.* **2021**, *47*, 487–502. [CrossRef]
10. Zhao, M.M.; Liu, B.H.; Wang, L.; Wu, Q.H.; Kang, Z.; Hao, Y.H.; Amporfro, D.; Gao, L.J. A Cross-Sectional Study on China's Public Health Emergency Personnel's Field Coping-Capacity: Need, Influencing Factors, and Improvement Options. *Disaster Med. Public Health Prep.* **2020**, *14*, 192–200. [CrossRef]
11. Chen, C.L.; Tang, J.S.; Lai, M.K.; Hung, C.H. Factors influencing medical staff's intentions to implement family-witnessed cardiopulmonary resuscitation: A cross-sectional, multihospital survey. *Eur. J. Cardiovasc. Nursing.* **2017**, *16*, 492–501. [CrossRef]
12. Rottger, S.; Maier, J.; Krex-Brinkmann, L.; Kowalski, J.T.; Krick, A.; Felfe, J.; Stein, M. Social cognitive aspects of the participation in workplace health promotion as revealed by the theory of planned behavior. *Prev. Med.* **2017**, *105*, 104–108. [CrossRef]
13. Rich, A.; Medisauskaite, A.; Potts, H.W.W.; Griffin, A. A theory-based study of doctors' intentions to engage in professional behaviours. *BMC Med. Educ.* **2020**, *20*, 44. [CrossRef]
14. Ajzen, I. The theory of planned behavior. *Organ. Behav. Hum. Decis. Process.* **1991**, *50*, 179–211. [CrossRef]
15. Bagozzi, R.P.; Dholakia, U.M.; Mookerjee, A. Individual and Group Bases of Social Influence in Online Environments. *Media Psychol.* **2006**, *8*, 95–126. [CrossRef]
16. Ajzen, I. The theory of planned behaviour: Reactions and reflections. *Psychol. Health* **2011**, *26*, 1113–1127. [CrossRef]
17. Malik, N.; Dhar, R.L. Authentic leadership and its impact on extra role behaviour of nurses: The mediating role of psychological capital and the moderating role of autonomy. *Pers. Rev.* **2017**, *46*, 277–296. [CrossRef]
18. Luthans, F.; Luthans, K.W.; Luthans, B.C. Positive psychological capital: Beyond human and social capital. *Bus. Horiz.* **2004**, *47*, 45–50. [CrossRef]
19. Seligman, M.E.P.; Csikszentmihalyi, M. Positive psychology: An introduction. *Am. Psychol.* **2000**, *55*, 5–14. [CrossRef] [PubMed]
20. Burns, A.J.; Posey, C.; Roberts, T.L.; Lowry, P.B. Examining the relationship of organizational insiders' psychological capital with information security threat and coping appraisals. *Comput. Hum. Behav.* **2017**, *68*, 190–209. [CrossRef]
21. Stratman, J.L.; Youssef-Morgan, C.M. Can positivity promote safety? Psychological capital development combats cynicism and unsafe behavior. *Saf. Sci.* **2019**, *116*, 13–25. [CrossRef]
22. Luthans, F.; Avey, J.B.; Avolio, B.J.; Norman, S.M.; Combs, G. Psychological Capital Development: Toward a Micro-intervention. *J. Organ. Behav.* **2006**, *27*, 387–393. [CrossRef]
23. Wang, J.F.; Bu, L.R.; Li, Y.; Song, J.; Li, N. The mediating effect of academic engagement between psychological capital and academic burnout among nursing students during the COVID-19 pandemic: A cross-sectional study. *Nurse Educ. Today* **2021**, *102*, 104938. [CrossRef] [PubMed]
24. Luthans, F.; Broad, J.D. Positive psychological capital to help combat the mental health fallout from the pandemic and VUCA environment. *Organ. Dyn.* **2020**, 100817. [CrossRef]
25. Dwyer, P.A.; Revell, S.M.H.; Sethares, K.A.; Ayotte, B.J. The influence of psychological capital, authentic leadership in preceptors, and structural empowerment on new graduate nurse burnout and turnover intent. *Appl. Nurs. Res.* **2019**, *48*, 37–44. [CrossRef]
26. Ahayalimudin, N.; Osman, N.N.S. Disaster management: Emergency nursing and medical personnel's knowledge, attitude and practices of the East Coast region hospitals of Malaysia. *Australas. Emerg. Nurs. J. AENJ* **2016**, *19*, 203–209. [CrossRef] [PubMed]
27. O'Boyle, C.; Robertson, C.; Secor-Turner, M. Nurses' beliefs about public health emergencies: Fear of abandonment. *Am. J. Infect. Control.* **2006**, *34*, 351–357. [CrossRef] [PubMed]
28. Via-Clavero, G.; Guardia-Olmos, J.; Falco-Pegueroles, A.; Gil-Castillejos, D.; Lobo-Civico, A.; De La Cueva-Ariza, L.; Romero-Garcia, M.; Delgado-Hito, P. Factors influencing critical care nurses' intentions to use physical restraints adopting the theory of planned behaviour: A cross-sectional multicentre study. *Aust. Crit. Care* **2020**, *33*, 426–435. [CrossRef]

29. Knowles, S.; Lam, L.T.; McInnes, E.; Elliott, D.; Hardy, J.; Middleton, S. Knowledge, attitudes, beliefs and behaviour intentions for three bowel management practices in intensive care: Effects of a targeted protocol implementation for nursing and medical staff. *BMC Nurs.* **2015**, *14*, 6. [CrossRef]
30. Corace, K.M.; Srigley, J.A.; Hargadon, D.P.; Yu, D.; MacDonald, T.K.; Fabrigar, L.R.; Garber, G.E. Using behavior change frameworks to improve healthcare worker influenza vaccination rates: A systematic review. *Vaccine* **2016**, *34*, 3235–3242. [CrossRef]
31. Lai, M.K.; Aritejo, B.A.; Tang, J.S.; Chen, C.L.; Chuang, C.C. Predicting medical professionals' intention to allow family presence during resuscitation: A cross sectional survey. *Int. J. Nurs. Stud.* **2017**, *70*, 11–16. [CrossRef]
32. Ghaffari, M.; Rakhshanderou, S.; Safari-Moradabadi, A.; Barkati, H. Exploring determinants of hand hygiene among hospital nurses: A qualitative study. *BMC Nurs.* **2020**, *19*, 109. [CrossRef]
33. Armitage, C.J.; Conner, M. Distinguishing Perceptions of Control from Self-Efficacy: Predicting Consumption of a Low-Fat Diet Using the Theory of Planned Behavior. *J. Appl. Soc. Psychol.* **2009**, *39*, 72–90. [CrossRef]
34. Paek, H.J.; Hilyard, K.; Freimuth, V.; Barge, J.K.; Mindlin, M. Theory-Based Approaches to Understanding Public Emergency Preparedness: Implications for Effective Health and Risk Communication. *J. Health Commun.* **2010**, *15*, 428–444. [CrossRef]
35. Al Khalaileh, M.A.; Bond, E.; Alasad, J.A. Jordanian nurses' perceptions of their preparedness for disaster management. *Int. Emerg. Nurs.* **2012**, *20*, 14–23. [CrossRef] [PubMed]
36. Boldor, N.; Br-Dayan, Y.; Rosenbloom, T.; Shemer, J.; Bar-Dayan, Y. Optimism of health care workers during a disaster: A review of the literature. *Emerg. Health Threat. J.* **2012**, *5*, 7270. [CrossRef] [PubMed]
37. Melnikov, S.; Itzhaki, M.; Kagan, I. Israeli Nurses' Intention to Report for Work in an Emergency or Disaster. *J. Nurs. Scholarsh.* **2014**, *46*, 134–142. [CrossRef]
38. Mache, S.; Vitzthum, K.; Wanke, E.; Groneberg, D.A.; Klapp, B.F.; Danzer, G. Exploring the impact of resilience, self-efficacy, optimism and organizational resources on work engagement. *WORK-A J. Prev. Assess. Rehabil.* **2014**, *47*, 491–500.
39. McAllister, S.; Coxon, K.; Murrells, T.; Sandall, J. Healthcare professionals' attitudes, knowledge and self-efficacy levels regarding the use of self-hypnosis in childbirth: A prospective questionnaire survey. *Midwifery* **2017**, *47*, 8–14. [CrossRef]
40. Tang, N.; Han, L.; Yang, P.; Zhao, Y.; Zhang, H. Are mindfulness and self-efficacy related to presenteeism among primary medical staff: A cross-sectional study. *Int. J. Nurs. Sci.* **2019**, *6*, 182–186. [CrossRef]
41. Nowakowska, I.; Rasinska, R.; Glowacka, M.D. The influence of factors of work environment and burnout syndrome on self-efficacy of medical staff. *Ann. Agric. Environ. Med.* **2016**, *23*, 304–309. [CrossRef]
42. Wu, L.F.; Chang, L.F.; Hung, Y.C.; Lin, C.; Tzou, S.J.; Chou, L.J.; Pan, H.H. The Effect of Practice toward Do-Not-Resuscitate among Taiwanese Nursing Staff Using Path Modeling. *Int. J. Environ. Res. Public Health* **2020**, *17*, 6350. [CrossRef] [PubMed]
43. Klaver, M.; van den Hoofdakker, B.J.; Wouters, H.; de Kuijper, G.; Hoekstra, P.J.; de Bildt, A. Exposure to challenging behaviours and burnout symptoms among care staff: The role of psychological resources. *J. Intellect. Disabil. Res.* **2021**, *65*, 173–185. [CrossRef] [PubMed]
44. Frey, R.; Robinson, J.; Wong, C.; Gott, M. Burnout, compassion fatigue and psychological capital: Findings from a survey of nurses delivering palliative care. *Appl. Nurs. Res.* **2018**, *43*, 1–9. [CrossRef]
45. Ajzen, I. Perceived Behavioral Control, Self-Efficacy, Locus of Control, and the Theory of Planned Behavior. *J. Appl. Soc. Psychol.* **2002**, *32*, 665–683. [CrossRef]
46. Probst, T.M.; Gailey, N.J.; Jiang, L.X.; Bohle, S.L. Psychological capital: Buffering the longitudinal curvilinear effects of job insecurity on performance. *Saf. Sci.* **2017**, *100*, 74–82. [CrossRef]
47. Liu, Y.; Aungsuroch, Y.; Gunawan, J.; Zeng, D.J. Job Stress, Psychological Capital, Perceived Social Support, and Occupational Burnout Among Hospital Nurses. *J. Nurs. Scholarsh.* **2021**, *53*, 511–518. [CrossRef]
48. Yildiz, H. The Interactive Effect of Positive Psychological Capital and Organizational Trust on Organizational Citizenship Behavior. *SAGE Open* **2019**, *9*, 1–15. [CrossRef]
49. Luthans, F.; Avolio, B.J.; Avey, J.B.; Norman, S.M. Positive Psychological Capital: Measurement and Relationship with Performance and Satisfaction. *Pers. Psychol.* **2007**, *60*, 541–572. [CrossRef]
50. Ajzen, I. Constructing a TPB Questionnaire: Conceptual and Methodological Considerations. *Work. Pap.* **2006**. Available online: http://www.people.umass.edu/aizen/pdf/tpb.measurement.pdf (accessed on 27 June 2021).
51. Miceli, R.; Sotgiu, I.; Settanni, M. Disaster preparedness and perception of flood risk: A study in an alpine valley in Italy. *J. Environ. Psychol.* **2008**, *28*, 164–173. [CrossRef]
52. Murphy, S.T.; Cody, M.; Frank, L.B.; Glik, D.; Ang, A. Predictors of emergency preparedness and compliance. *Disaster Med. Public Health Prep.* **2009**, *7*, S1–S8. [CrossRef] [PubMed]
53. Hong, Y.X.; Kim, J.S.; Xiong, L.H. Media exposure and individuals' emergency preparedness behaviors for coping with natural and human-made disasters. *J. Environ. Psychol.* **2019**, *63*, 82–91. [CrossRef]
54. Kohn, S.; Eaton, J.L.; Feroz, S.; Bainbridge, A.A.; Hoolachan, J.; Barnett, D.J. Personal Disaster Preparedness: An Integrative Review of the Literature. *Disaster Med. Public Health Prep.* **2012**, *6*, 217–231. [CrossRef]
55. McNeill, C.C.; Killian, T.S.; Moon, Z.; Way, K.A.; Betsy Garrison, M.E. The Relationship Between Perceptions of Emergency Preparedness, Disaster Experience, Health-Care Provider Education, and Emergency Preparedness Levels. *Int. Q. Community Health Educ.* **2018**, *38*, 233–243. [CrossRef]

56. Ndu, A.C.; Kassy, W.C.; Ochie, C.N.; Arinze-Onyia, S.U.; Okeke, T.A.; Aguwa, E.N.; Okwor, T.J.; Chinawa, A. Knowledge, Misperceptions, Preparedness, and Barriers towards Lassa Fever Control among Health Care Workers in a Tertiary Institution in Enugu, Nigeria. *J. Health Care Poor Underserved* **2019**, *30*, 1151–1164. [CrossRef] [PubMed]
57. Taylor, A.B.; MacKinnon, D.P.; Tein, J.Y. Tests of the three-path mediated effect. *Organ. Res. Methods* **2008**, *11*, 241–269. [CrossRef]
58. Biesanz, J.C.; Falk, C.F.; Savalei, V. Assessing Mediational Models: Testing and Interval Estimation for Indirect Effects. *Multivar. Behav. Res.* **2010**, *45*, 661–701. [CrossRef] [PubMed]
59. Yin, Y. Characteristics of Social Governing Organizations and Governance of Emergent Public Security Events from the Perspective of Public Safety. *Rev. De Cercet. Interv. Soc.* **2020**, *69*, 241–260.

MDPI
St. Alban-Anlage 66
4052 Basel
Switzerland
Tel. +41 61 683 77 34
Fax +41 61 302 89 18
www.mdpi.com

International Journal of Environmental Research and Public Health Editorial Office
E-mail: ijerph@mdpi.com
www.mdpi.com/journal/ijerph

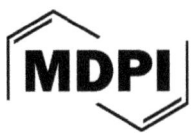